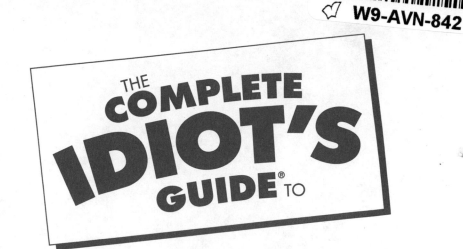

THE
COMPLETE
IDIOT'S
GUIDE® TO

Sleep Training for Your Child

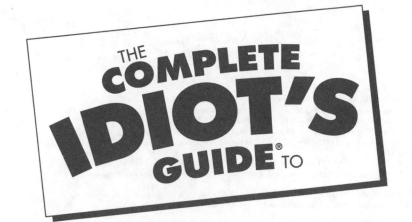

THE
COMPLETE
IDIOT'S
GUIDE® TO

Sleep Training
for Your Child

*by Melissa Burnham, Ph.D.
and Jennifer Lawler, Ph.D.*

ALPHA

A Member of Penguin Group (USA) Inc.

To Nickolas—MB
To Jessica—JL

ALPHA BOOKS

Published by the Penguin Group

Penguin Group (USA) Inc., 375 Hudson Street, New York, New York 10014, U.S.A.

Penguin Group (Canada), 10 Alcorn Avenue, Toronto, Ontario, Canada M4V 3B2 (a division of Pearson Penguin Canada Inc.)

Penguin Books Ltd, 80 Strand, London WC2R 0RL, England

Penguin Ireland, 25 St Stephen's Green, Dublin 2, Ireland (a division of Penguin Books Ltd)

Penguin Group (Australia), 250 Camberwell Road, Camberwell, Victoria 3124, Australia (a division of Pearson Australia Group Pty Ltd)

Penguin Books India Pvt Ltd, 11 Community Centre, Panchsheel Park, New Delhi—110 017, India

Penguin Group (NZ), cnr Airborne and Rosedale Roads, Albany, Auckland 1310, New Zealand (a division of Pearson New Zealand Ltd)

Penguin Books (South Africa) (Pty) Ltd, 24 Sturdee Avenue, Rosebank, Johannesburg 2196, South Africa

Penguin Books Ltd, Registered Offices: 80 Strand, London WC2R 0RL, England

Copyright © 2006 by Melissa Burnham, Ph.D. and Jennifer Lawler, Ph.D.

International Standard Book Number: 1-59257-540-4
Library of Congress Catalog Card Number: 2006903505

08   07   06   8   7   6   5   4   3   2   1

Interpretation of the printing code: The rightmost number of the first series of numbers is the year of the book's printing; the rightmost number of the second series of numbers is the number of the book's printing. For example, a printing code of 06-1 shows that the first printing occurred in 2006.

Printed in the United States of America

Note: This publication contains the opinions and ideas of its authors. It is intended to provide helpful and informative material on the subject matter covered. It is sold with the understanding that the authors and publisher are not engaged in rendering professional services in the book. If the reader requires personal assistance or advice, a competent professional should be consulted.

The authors and publisher specifically disclaim any responsibility for any liability, loss, or risk, personal or otherwise, which is incurred as a consequence, directly or indirectly, of the use and application of any of the contents of this book.

Most Alpha books are available at special quantity discounts for bulk purchases for sales promotions, premiums, fund-raising, or educational use. Special books, or book excerpts, can also be created to fit specific needs.

For details, write: Special Markets, Alpha Books, 375 Hudson Street, New York, NY 10014.

Publisher: *Marie Butler-Knight*
Editorial Director: *Mike Sanders*
Managing Editor: *Billy Fields*
Acquisitions Editor: *Tom Stevens*
Development Editor: *Michael Thomas*
Production Editor: *Megan Douglass*
Copy Editor: *Jan Zoya*

Cover Designer: *Bill Thomas*
Book Designers: *Trina Wurst/Kurt Owens*
Indexer: *Julie Bess*
Layout: *Chad Dressler*
Proofreader: *Aaron Black*

Contents at a Glance

Contents

Foreword

Sleep. That blissful yet sometimes elusive state of being that rejuvenates our tired bodies, recharges our over-taxed brains, and re-energizes our spirits. The lack thereof which leads to cranky mornings, fuzzy afternoons, and (with apologies to Walt Disney) the "sleepy/dopey/grumpy syndrome." Not to mention the consumption of alarming amounts of high-octane, highly caffeinated specialty beverages.

Sleeping like a baby. The very phrase conjures up visions of peaceful slumber, effortlessly restful nights, and rosy-cheeked, feetie-pajama-clad cherubs drifting off to Dreamland, clutching blankies in their chubby fists. But what if "sleeping like a baby" in *your* house instead translates to bitter bedtime battles, midnight howls, endless hours spent in a rocking chair, and flat-out total exhaustion when the alarm rings at 6 A.M.?

Buck up, bleary-eyed Moms and Dads, help is on the way! *The Complete Idiot's Guide to Sleep Training for Your Child* is the perfect antidote to the baby bedtime blues. Chockfull of sage, well-grounded, and *practical* advice, this book will provide you with all you need to know to solve your child's sleep woes, *your* way.

But "*sleep training*," you say? Isn't that something you might do with a recalcitrant puppy, not your precious little bundle of joy? In fact, sleep training is a perfectly legitimate term we behavioral psychology–minded types use to describe the process of teaching a child to fall asleep naturally and easily, and to stay asleep through the night. That's right, *teach*. Because like taking those first wobbly steps, mastering a sippy cup, and riding a bicycle, sleeping is an instinctive yet complex process that is two parts nature, one part nurture, and the rest learned behavior. And there are almost as many choices of sleep instruction methods out there as there are unhappy babies on the block.

So what's a tired, easily confused, and, let's face it, not exactly rational at 3 A.M. parent to do? Unlike other sleep manuals out there, *The Complete Idiot's Guide to Sleep Training for Your Child* provides information and how-to's for *all* the major sleep problem-solving techniques, from the "cry it out/ignore it" approach to the "Ferber/ignore but check" method to the "scheduled awakenings," "persistent gentle removal," and "wait it out" systems, rather than advocating a specific one-size-fits-all plan. *The Complete Idiot's Guide to Sleep Training for Your Child* will help you match a sleep training method to your "parenting philosophy" and family's lifestyle by exploring all the common challenges and pitfalls, outlining pros and cons, and providing in-the-trenches feedback from parents who have tried the various approaches.

Painstakingly step-by-step, the book includes troubleshooting tips, as well as pointers for special circumstances (i.e., older and special needs children, colicky babies, and so on.). It also covers all the ABC's of ZZZ's, ranging from normal sleep development, sleep needs, and sleep hygiene, to bedtime routines, napping, and sleep schedules, while emphasizing good, healthy sleep habits for the *whole* family, *including* parents. Never preachy, it includes an intelligent and fair-minded discussion of bed-sharing pluses and minuses, and even covers hypnosis, meditation, guided imagery, Yoga, massage, swaddling, and Tai Chi methods for soothing the savage baby.

So take heart, frazzled fellow parents; down that last swallow of double espresso latte, and read on. You are about to enter the wonderful world of dream-filled nights and sun-drenched, happy days. Your baby (and your boss) will thank you for it, 'cause if baby ain't happy, ain't nobody happy. Good night and good luck.

—Judith Owens, M.D., Director, Pediatric Sleep Disorders Clinic, Hasbro Children's Hospital, Providence, Rhode Island

Introduction

We hate to break it to you, but if you have a baby (or are about to get one), sooner or later you'll encounter sleep problems. Actually, your baby will encounter the sleep problems … but if baby ain't happy, nobody's happy. It might be that you have trouble getting your little one to fall asleep at bedtime, or he might wake repeatedly at night and not be able to get back to sleep without help from you, or you might be one of the lucky ones whose child has both problems.

A recent study conducted at Brown University Medical School showed that the majority of children (including babies) do not get enough sleep—and lack of sleep causes many problems, including mood swings, irritability, and difficulty focusing.

If your baby or child has trouble sleeping, you'll have trouble sleeping. That sleep deprivation is what pushes most parents to try to sleep train their babies—the parents just can't continue to function on not enough sleep. (Sure, the baby gets to nap! But you have work to do.)

That's why this book can help. We'll show you what you need to know about how babies and children sleep—including how much they should sleep. Because many older children who have sleep problems had them when they were younger, we'd encourage you to start addressing sleep problems when your child is young—but not a newborn!

No matter if your child is young or old, you'll find *The Complete Idiot's Guide to Sleep Training for Your Child* full of information that can help you and your baby get some sleep.

What's in the Book?

The Complete Idiot's Guide to Sleep Training for Your Child is divided into five parts, and each part covers a different area of sleep training. You can read it from start to finish, or you can turn directly to the information you need most.

In **Part 1, "Sleep 101,"** we answer questions like "What *is* sleep training?" and "How many methods are there?" This part of the book introduces you to the idea of sleep training your baby or child, and gives you the lowdown on how to create a method to the madness.

In **Part 2, "Crying It Out,"** we discover that sometimes the best way to help your baby is to … not help her. In this part, we'll show the various "cry it out" sleep-training methods, also called "extinction" methods. We'll explain why letting your baby cry (not all night, of course) can help your baby learn to fall asleep and learn how to fall back to sleep after night wakings.

If the idea of letting your sweet baby cry at night is more than you can bear, you'll probably want to try a kinder, gentler approach. In **Part 3, "No More Tears,"** we'll explain several different sleep-training methods that don't require you to let your baby cry while you ignore him.

Maybe you got a bargain with your baby—she learned to fall asleep at night with no troubles and quickly picked up on self-soothing techniques so that she could get herself back to sleep after night wakings. But now that she's older, bedtime has become a battleground. Or maybe your child has always had sleep issues and you are now feeling the need to deal with them. What to do? In **Part 4, "My Baby's Not a Baby! Sleep Training for Children,"** we'll show how to use sleep-training approaches with toddlers and children young and old. We'll help you figure out which approach to try, and we'll explain why children have sleep problems that babies don't.

You know how a spa day makes you feel good all over? Well, some of the same techniques—massage, yoga, and soothing music—can be used with your little one to help him fall asleep. In **Part 5, "Holistic and New-Age Approaches,"** we'll show you how to find the right approach for you and your baby and explain how to integrate it with other sleep-training approaches.

Extras

You'll also find additional information, research results, anecdotes, and tips about sleep training your child in little boxes throughout the book. Here's what they are:

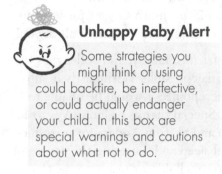

Unhappy Baby Alert

Some strategies you might think of using could backfire, be ineffective, or could actually endanger your child. In this box are special warnings and cautions about what not to do.

Melissa's Mindset

Want to know if the promises a sleep-training approach makes are scientifically accurate? Here you'll find the lowdown on the research that has been conducted and what it says about various sleep-training claims. We'll also reveal Melissa's thoughts, experiences, and reactions to sleep-training claims.

Infant Almanac

Tidbits, facts, and statistics about sleep training that help you understand what's up with your baby or child.

BABY BABBLE

Does sleep researcher-ese leave you baffled? Here, you'll find jargon and expressions related to sleep training defined. Definitions can also be found in the glossary.

Acknowledgments

We'd like to thank our agent, Marilyn Allen, for all her hard work. Our editor at *Complete Idiot's Guides*, Tom Stevens, is a dream to work with. We'd also like to thank our technical reviewer, Lisa Meltzer, who made sure we didn't make any egregious mistakes. We also appreciate all the parents who shared their stories of what sleep-training methods did—and didn't—work for them. Thanks to Judith Owens for writing the foreword to our book. We couldn't have done it without all of you!

Melissa would also like to thank the friends, family, and colleagues (you know who you are!) who make every day possible. Without their support, friendship, and unconditional acceptance, I would be unable to pursue fun projects such as this one. Special thanks to James Wyatt for introducing me to sleep 15 years ago and to Tom Anders for introducing me to the world of developmental sleep and sculpting the course of my work. Last but not least, thanks to Nickolas for teaching me that research and real life can coincide.

Jennifer would also like to give a shout out to her freelancing buddies who help her stay sane (or at least as sane as she's likely to be).

Trademarks

All terms mentioned in this book that are known to be or are suspected of being trademarks or service marks have been appropriately capitalized. Alpha Books and Penguin Group (USA) Inc. cannot attest to the accuracy of this information. Use of a term in this book should not be regarded as affecting the validity of any trademark or service mark.

1

Sleep 101

You've got the baby and you've finally got the hang of this diapering business. You can feed her and dress her and even bathe her. But you can't get her to sleep. What do you do? We're here to help.

This part of the book shows you what sleep training is, gives you an idea of what the various schools of thought are, and helps you compare the methods so that soon your baby will be sleeping like a baby.

Chapter 1

What Is Sleep Training?

In This Chapter

- ◆ Understanding what sleep training is
- ◆ Practicing safe sleeping
- ◆ Why you may want to try sleep training
- ◆ Making order out of chaos
- ◆ Planning your responses instead of reacting to sleep problems

In this chapter, we'll give you the lowdown on what sleep training is. We'll show why you might consider using one of the sleep-training methods we describe in this book to help your baby (or your older child) learn to fall asleep (and to fall back to sleep after waking at night) without too many problems—at least in the long run. In the short run, sleep training takes time, patience, and persistence.

We'll also describe the basic differences between the main approaches to sleep training so that you can make the right decision about how (and even if) you should sleep train your baby or child.

Training Who?

Sleep training is, simply put, using specific, proven strategies to help your baby ...

- ◆ Learn to fall asleep by himself at bedtime.

- ◆ Learn to fall back to sleep when she wakes during the night.

All babies wake during the night until they're at least 1 or 2 years old; some just learn to go back to sleep without help from their caretakers. We're betting that you probably want to have one of those children who can fall back to sleep without help.

> **Infant Almanac**
>
> In Parts 2 and 3, we'll cover in step-by-step detail how to use the various sleep-training approaches—everything from "ignoring it" (also known as "crying it out") to using the family bed. In Part 4, we show how these methods can be used for toddlers through preteens.

> **BABY BABBLE**
>
> **Self-soothing** is the ability of a baby or child to comfort herself after waking without requiring parental presence (feeding, rocking, etc.).

Many of the approaches that we'll present focus on teaching your baby *self-soothing* methods so that your presence is not required for him to fall asleep or to fall back asleep. Others assume that you'll be present when your baby needs to get to sleep. Which route you choose depends on a variety of factors, many of which we describe later in this chapter.

Even though the goal of sleep training is to train your baby (or child), in most cases, you'll have to train yourself, too! That means when you decide to try a sleep-training approach, you need to be sure that you're willing to do what needs to be done, and to follow through with the required steps. If there's a problem with your child's sleep, inconsistency on your part will only make it worse.

Ensuring Safe Sleep

No matter what you decide to do about sleep training your baby—and even if you decide not to sleep train her at all—you'll want to ensure that your baby sleeps safely.

"Back to sleep" is the phrase to remember when it comes time to put your baby down to sleep. The risk of Sudden Infant Death Syndrome (SIDS) is dramatically reduced when babies are placed on their backs to sleep.

The cause of SIDS is unclear; it probably has several causes. However, studies have shown that SIDS deaths can be cut in half by putting babies to sleep on their backs. This is most important in the first few months of the baby's life when the risk of SIDS is highest. Once the baby can easily roll from back to front (and the reverse) on his own, there is no need to fret about positioning.

Melissa's Mindset

Sometimes pediatricians recommend "sidelying" (putting baby to bed on her side) for babies who spit up a lot. Make sure that you understand exactly how to position your baby if this is recommended for her. Most pediatricians now recommend putting baby on her back to sleep, as does the American Academy of Pediatrics.

Babies do need to spend time on their tummies—otherwise they'll take longer to learn to crawl and develop other crucial physical skills. They can also develop a flattened head if left mostly on their backs. So you need to place baby on her tummy on the floor while you play with her and supervise her during the day. This "tummy time" is very important for the baby to develop the strong back muscles necessary for appropriate motor development.

Here are some other sleep safety precautions to take:

◆ Avoid soft bedding, which can cause suffocation. Infants under 12 months should sleep in a one-piece sleeper with no pillows or blankets in the crib.

Infant Almanac

Let's say you put your baby on his back to sleep—but he rolls over. What should you do? According to the American Academy of Pediatrics, by the time a baby can roll over, the highest risk of SIDS has passed, so you probably don't need to worry about it. But consult your physician if you're concerned about the situation or if your baby has problems such as sleep apnea that increase his risk of SIDS.

Unhappy Baby Alert

The National Safety Council website has additional information on precautions that can help keep your baby sleeping safely. See www.nsc.org for more in formation.

♦ Spaces between crib slats should be no wider than 2 ⅜ inches— otherwise your baby's head could be trapped. Be extremely cautious of used or antique cribs. Also avoid cribs with decorative cutouts in the headboard or footboard.

♦ Place a firm mattress in the crib.

♦ Eliminate spaces between the mattress and crib walls.

♦ Never put your baby to sleep on a waterbed, pillow, sofa, or other soft surface.

♦ Don't place a rolled-up towel or similar item in the crib to keep the baby from rolling over.

♦ Keep the room temperature cool, around 65–70°.

You'll want to take additional special precautions if you plan to use the "family bed" (also called "co-sleeping") approach. See Chapter 12 for more information on safely sharing a bed with your baby or child.

Why Sleep Train?

If you have to ask, you probably haven't had a newborn in the house lately. If your baby sleeps poorly, so do you. Even worse, your baby may be fussy and hard to soothe if she doesn't get enough sleep. Overtired babies are cranky babies! Because of sleep deprivation, you (and any other adult sharing nighttime duty) may become more anxious, depressed, and irritable, not to mention drowsy and lacking in focus.

In addition, teaching your baby good sleep habits now helps him stay happy and healthy and will be a good basis for healthy sleep habits throughout childhood. Studies show that children who have sleep problems have usually had them since infancy. One study showed that nearly 85 percent of 3-year-olds had had sleep problems since they were born! If you don't want your baby to become a statistic (that is, a child with sleep problems), then you may want to sleep train him now.

If your baby isn't a baby, you might be tired of constant night wakings that interrupt your sleep and sap your patience. For older babies and children, sleep training can help them sleep through the night and wake refreshed and ready the next morning. By getting serious about sleep training, you can ensure that everyone in the family gets enough shut-eye to do well the next day.

Creating a Method to the Madness

Most sleep-training approaches encourage some essential methods to put a lid on the chaos, such as the following:

◆ Creating a basic schedule for your daily life

◆ Helping your new baby distinguish night from day

◆ Creating a relaxing bedtime routine for your child (and yourself!)

◆ Encouraging good sleep habits in your child

Infant Almanac

No matter which sleep-training approach you choose, getting started by keeping a more regular schedule and developing a bed-time routine will help you make order out of chaos!

Melissa's Mindset

Babies can't—and shouldn't—be strictly sleep trained until at least 6 months of age. That doesn't mean you can't instill some good habits very early (such as helping baby understand the difference between night and day, creating bedtime routines, and sticking to a reasonable schedule). But the stricter "ignoring" methods should not be attempted before the baby is at least 6 months old.

By developing a method to cope with the erratic sleep schedules of most babies, you can start your child on the road to good sleep habits.

Planning Versus Reacting

Many parents find themselves responding reactively to the sleep problems their babies and children experience. For example, the baby cries a lot, so they bring her to bed with them when she's most sleep deprived. It's not a planned strategy, just a reaction to a problem. But it can create another problem: a child who won't sleep in her own bed at night. And it doesn't solve the problem of why the child has trouble falling asleep in the first place.

On the other hand, if you *plan* to have your baby in bed with you, you're being proactive, and that's just fine. Snuggling with your little one is just all part of the master plan.

> **Infant Almanac**
>
> The best bet is for you to decide how you're going to sleep train your baby or child to get a good night's sleep. Planning puts you in control and will probably result in better sleep habits for your baby.

If you're just starting out on this journey toward parenthood and haven't had your child yet, try to keep a flexible mindset with regard to planning how you will deal with the baby's sleep. Some parents think they will be co-sleepers; others think they will be strict "cry it out" followers. Often, once the baby arrives, the plan changes, depending on the baby himself and how the parents now feel with the little one in arm. Just try to remain flexible with your thinking so that you can find the best way for all of you to get some shut-eye.

Being a Good Role Model

Don't forget that one of the best ways you can keep some sanity with a new baby in the house is to take care of yourself. Make sure you keep a regular schedule (including on weekends), get enough rest, and get help with your baby as you need it. See Chapter 5 for more information on taking care of yourself even with a newborn in the house.

By setting a good example for your baby, you may be able to help encourage good sleep habits in her.

Understanding the Sleep Training Schools of Thought

Basically, two schools of thought regarding sleep training exist—we might call them "cry it out" versus "no more tears":

♦ Supporters of "cry it out" approaches feel that your baby shouldn't run the show—you should.

♦ Supporters of "no more tears" approaches feel that your parenting should be child-centered and that your responses should be guided by your child.

That's an over-simplification, of course, but it helps show the differences in the approaches. Between the most extreme methods—the abrupt "ignore it" approach and the "almost-anything-goes" child-centered approach—you'll find plenty of middle ground. It's in this middle ground that most parents find relief from their baby's sleep problems.

Infant Almanac

We can't stress enough the importance of understanding the method and being willing to follow it step-by-step. It is also important for your partner or other adult caretakers involved to agree to participate. Otherwise, you could make matters worse.

Infant Almanac

Be sure to show grandparents, other relatives, and all caretakers the best way to put your baby to sleep. Even if they put their babies to sleep on their tummies, insist on having everyone follow your rules. It's true that babies do sleep better on their tummies, but that's not the point. You want your baby to be able to wake up when faced with a life-threatening event. That's why back sleeping is recommended.

Many sleep-training approaches have been developed to solve one of the two specific sleep-training problems:

♦ Helping your baby fall asleep at bedtime

♦ Helping your baby fall back to sleep after night wakings

It's important to understand the distinction, because some of the approaches that focus on how you can get your baby to fall back to sleep after night wakings—such as the "scheduled awakenings" approach discussed in Chapter 10—won't be of any use to you if your problem is getting your baby to fall asleep in the first place.

In Chapter 4, we'll discuss how to pick the right sleep-training approach for you and your baby.

Crying It Out

The "crying it out" sleep-training approaches are referred to as "extinction" methods by sleep researchers. The process "extinguishes" or "puts out" the problem with firm and decisive action.

The basic idea behind these approaches is that if you ignore your baby's crying at bedtime, he will learn (eventually) to fall asleep without your intervention. Of course, you need to have strong nerves to ignore the crying baby!

On the most extreme end of the "cry it out" spectrum, you just pretty much ignore the crying until it stops, at which point your nerves will be mostly tattered. But less-abrupt approaches can also work out and are probably easier on most parents' nerves.

These less-abrupt approaches include methods that allow for checking on your baby, or that require you to gradually remove yourself from your baby's presence. We describe these "cry it out" approaches in Part 2 (Chapters 6–9).

Avoiding the Tears

For parents who can't imagine letting their baby cry it out—or who have tried such an approach but failed spectacularly—there are kinder, gentler approaches to try. The drawback is that these approaches may take longer to work, require more parental involvement, or could confuse the baby.

> **Infant Almanac**
>
> In Part 4 (Chapters 16–19), we show how to apply both types of approaches to toddlers, school-agers, preteens, and children with special needs.

In this category fall approaches such as "scheduled awakenings," where you do an end run around your baby's night wakings by waking *her* up before she can wake *you* up, to sharing the bed—the "family bed" or "co-sleeping" approach. These methods are described in Part 3 (Chapters 10–15).

Although these tear-free methods can seem very appealing to parents, sometimes they don't work as desired and the parent ends up choosing one of the extinction methods. This is especially true when parents get frustrated at how long it's taking for the method to work with their child—they're so sleep deprived that they need quicker results.

Complementary, Holistic, and New Age Approaches

Babies and children also respond to unconventional approaches to help them sleep, such as massage, yoga—even hypnosis. These "complementary" approaches, described in Part 5 (Chapters 20–22), aren't meant to replace traditional sleep-training methods—they complement them and are used in conjunction with them. These approaches help your child relax and feel ready to settle down for the night.

Deciding on Sleep-Training Goals

You've decided that you need to sleep train your baby or child. What's your next step? It should be deciding on your sleep-training goals.

If you don't know what you're hoping to accomplish, you may choose the wrong approach to sleep training, or you may find it difficult to remain committed to the method during challenges.

Responding true or false to the following statements can help you decide on sleep-training goals:

1. My baby's sleep habits are a problem for me.

   If true, then you need to determine why your baby's sleep habits are a problem (e.g., not settling down at night, or waking too frequently at night).

   If false, then you don't have a problem.

Melissa's Mindset

Make sure your goals and expectations are compatible with your child's abilities. It's unrealistic to think that a 1-month-old baby can sleep through the night. At the same time, don't underestimate the ability of your older baby to soothe herself back to sleep after a night waking.

2. My baby has trouble falling asleep at bedtime.

   If true, then you need to choose an approach that is designed to combat this problem (such as the "extinction" method described in Chapter 6).

   If false, then you need to decide what sleep problem your child has.

3. My baby has trouble with night wakings.

   If true, then you need to choose an approach that is designed to help solve this problem (such as the "scheduled awakenings" approach described in Chapter 10).

   If false, then you need to decide what sleep problem your child has.

4. My baby has both problems: trouble settling down for the night and waking frequently at night.

   If true, then decide whether you want to tackle both problems at the same time. If so, then choose the appropriate approach, such as the "graduated extinction" method described in Chapter 7. If no, then choose the "splitting it up" approach described in Chapter 9.

Once you know what you're trying to accomplish, you'll want to look at Chapter 4 to help you get started and then read about the various sleep-training approaches you can try.

The most important thing to keep in mind is that if the baby's sleep habits are not a problem for you or the baby, then there is no need to go to great lengths to change anything.

The Least You Need to Know

◆ Sleep training can help your baby or child develop good sleep habits so that everyone can get a good night's sleep.

◆ Despite the big differences in the various types of sleep-training approaches, developing a regular (yet flexible) schedule and a set bedtime routine can help everyone get some shut-eye.

◆ No matter what approach you choose, you need to make sure your baby sleeps safely.

◆ There's a sleep-training approach to suit every parent and child.

Chapter 2

Sleeping Like a Baby

In This Chapter

- ◆ Helping your baby learn to distinguish night from day
- ◆ Understanding how babies' sleep patterns develop over time
- ◆ Recognizing—and getting help for—sleep problems in your baby
- ◆ Understanding circadian rhythms
- ◆ Knowing what to expect with sleep frequency and duration through the first year

Babies really are different from you and me. In this chapter, we'll show you just how and why that little bundle of joy sleeps the way she does—or doesn't.

We'll also describe typical sleep patterns for babies from newborn to 1 year, and we'll give you some pointers on helping your baby start to appreciate the difference between night and day.

Why Babies Don't Know Night from Day

Your baby's sleep—and yours—is regulated by an inborn biological clock. The wake/sleep cycle is part of your baby's circadian rhythm (24-hour cycles that include metabolic function, hormonal secretions, and other body functions).

Although this rhythm is inborn, it takes time to develop. So newborns have very erratic sleep cycles (but you knew that because you haven't slept for the last month).

At about 4 to 6 weeks of age, the baby's sleep-wake circadian rhythm *begins* to develop. Your baby won't have a regular sleep/wake cycle until about 4 to 6 months. The cycle may not resemble yours, but it will follow a 24-hour pattern. (The less the cycle resembles yours, the more likely it will seem to be a problem to you.)

Infant Almanac

Your baby's circadian rhythm—and sleep cycle—is set to local time. Your baby's body can reset the cycle but it can take a few days for that to occur. So if, for example, you travel with your baby, you'll find that he's sleeping according to the time zone you left, not the time zone you're in. If you're only going to be gone a few days, it's probably best to keep your baby on "home" time rather than transitioning him to the new clock time only to have to immediately transition him back again.

Melissa's Mindset

When researchers measure babies' sleep objectively, some find that babies are actually sleeping more at night than during the day from the very first weeks of life. Although a researcher might be able to measure a significant difference, for the most part parents won't notice a strong differentiation between night and daytime sleep until about four months.

While your baby's cycle will eventually include longer sleep periods, he doesn't necessarily know night from day. That's right: your baby has to *learn* the difference between night and day.

So those longer sleep periods might happen in the middle of the day, instead of at night, as you would probably prefer. By about 4 months, many babies are adapted to a day/night schedule, sleeping more at night than during the day.

To encourage your baby to distinguish night from day, try the following:

◆ Keep night feedings calm and quiet. Put your baby back to bed as soon as he has finished eating.

◆ Keep the baby's room dark at night.

◆ Expose the baby to light (especially sunlight) during the day.

◆ Play with the baby more during the day. Keeping him stimulated during daytime hours will help him recognize that nighttime is for sleeping.

◆ Wake her for feeding during the day, even if she is sleeping soundly.

◆ Be a loudmouth. During the day, make no special effort to keep the noise down. Your baby will learn that day is for activities and night is for sleep.

◆ Breastfeed naturally at night. Breastfeeding moms sometimes express milk during the day to feed to their babies at night because it's a way to get their partner involved in nighttime feedings. However, babies get an important nighttime signal through breast milk—their mother's melatonin (a hormone that aids sleep). Melatonin is secreted only at night. If you express during the day to feed at night, your baby is missing an important nighttime signal.

Melissa's Mindset

When doing a small research study on the development of circadian rhythms in babies, I was surprised to find that many parents used a bright light during the nighttime for changing or feeding the baby. The babies whose parents regularly used a bright light developed circadian rhythms later than those whose parents kept it relatively dark at night.

Connecting the Dots Between Feeding and Sleeping

New babies eat, sleep, and cry (and they fill up diapers pretty well, too). These activities are connected to one another: the baby cries because she's hungry or tired; she sleeps when she's full.

Infant Almanac

Breastfed babies do need to be fed slightly more often than formula-fed babies and they are more prone to night wakings, especially at first. Believe it or not, waking more often is actually thought to be a good thing for your baby, especially during the period when Sudden Infant Death Syndrome (SIDS) most frequently occurs. (See Chapter 1 for more information on SIDS.)

But it's important not to place too strong an emphasis on any connection between sleeping and feeding. Yes, your baby is more likely to fall asleep and stay asleep if her tummy is full, but feeding solids to a baby to help fill her tummy doesn't actually make her sleep better.

Your newborn baby will follow a wake-eat-play-sleep cycle every 2–3 hours at first. As he gets older, the time will lengthen and he'll go longer between feedings and will sleep for longer chunks of time (hopefully at night).

What Can You Expect?

Your friends may regale you with stories of babies who slept through the night right away—or they may scare you with tales from the dark side of babies who wouldn't sleep no matter what they tried.

There's no way of knowing which kind of baby you'll get, but the truth is, most babies don't sleep through the night (meaning something along the lines of falling asleep at midnight and waking again at 5 A.M.) until they're around 3 months old, and even that's not quite accurate: babies will wake throughout the night through the first year and beyond. Some babies just learn not to bother you about it. This is actually the point of sleep training: helping the baby/child to be able to fall back to sleep on her own after those inevitable awakenings.

Because babies may not sleep on their parents' schedule, it may seem like they're not sleeping much at all. But young babies do have an amazing capacity for sleep and in fact spend most of their time snoozing. As they grow older, they gradually spend more time awake. By the age of 1, most babies sleep about 13 hours out of every 24, divided between one or two daytime naps and nighttime sleep.

Your Baby's Sleep Needs

Babies sleep a lot. The following averages are just that—averages. Your baby may sleep more or less. If it's significantly more or less, you may want to consult your pediatrician or pediatric sleep specialist to rule out any problems.

- Newborn: 16–18 hours

- 1–3 months: 15–16 hours

- 3–6 months: 14–15 hours

- 6–12 months: 13–14 hours

- 1–2 years: 13 hours

- 2–3 years: 12 hours

- 3–5 years: 11 hours

Remember that these averages are across 24 hours, so they include both nighttime and daytime sleep.

Even at 1 year of age, most babies are still taking two naps per day. Most babies drop the second nap around 18 months. And most children continue to take one nap (usually an afternoon nap) every day through the third year of life. Some continue to need a nap or rest time every day through age 5. If your child is older than this and is still taking a daytime nap, you may wish to consult your pediatrician or a pediatric sleep specialist.

When Will This Baby Sleep Through the Night?

Most babies wake throughout the night until they're a year or two old. Some learn to put themselves back to sleep without needing any help from you.

Here is the approximate number of night wakings to expect per age:

◆ Up to 6 months: 2–3 wakings per night

◆ Up to 1 year: 1–2 wakings per night

◆ For some children, up to 2 years: 1–2 wakings per night

You can encourage your older baby to fall back to sleep without your help by using a sleep-training method designed for night wakings.

Colicky Babies

Most babies cry about 3 hours a day at 6 weeks of age, but fortunately not all at one time. They cry because they're hungry, tired, wet, bored, or just smacked themselves in the face with a flailing fist. But some babies cry way more than that and for reasons that are inexplicable. If your baby cries inconsolably for hours at a time, colic is likely the culprit.

Unhappy Baby Alert

About 20 percent of all babies develop colic. It's a little more common in first babies than in later babies, and it happens more with boys than girls.

Colic ordinarily does not develop until about 3 or 4 weeks of age and it usually goes away at about the age of 4 or 5 months. Generally the inconsolable crying happens in the afternoon or evening, and it lasts for 3 or more hours, for at least *3* days a week, for at least 3 weeks. After the crying episode, the baby stops and falls asleep, by which time the parents are crying themselves.

If your baby has colic, try the following:

◆ Check with your pediatrician to make sure there's no medical cause for the crying.

◆ Try swaddling your baby by wrapping her firmly in a blanket.

◆ Rub your baby's back.

◆ Sing or hum a low tune or play low, soothing music.

◆ Walk, rock, or ride in a car, or let baby swing in an infant swing.

◆ Feed the baby.

- Change the baby.

- Hold the baby.

- Let the baby suck (pacifier or her fingers).

- Warm the baby up—a warm blanket fresh from the dryer can soothe the baby.

- To avoid getting frustrated, trade off with a partner or another caretaker.

- Don't worry, be happy—you'll eventually become attuned to your baby and learn to distinguish her cries and understand what she wants (at least most of the time).

Melissa's Mindset

Despite the "common wisdom" dispersed by many well-intentioned neighbors and grandparents, there is no indication that colic is due to a gastrointestinal problem (gas) for most babies. Colic most commonly happens during the evening hours, which comes to be known by some parents as "the witching hour" (or 2 or 3). Mercifully, colic goes away on its own before most parents are driven to the point of insanity.

How Babies' Sleep Develops over Time

Everyone (including babies) experiences two types of sleep: REM and NREM.

- REM (rapid eye movement) is the active sleep during which you dream. In young infants, REM is referred to as "active sleep" because they flail around quite a bit and their eyes dart under their eyelids. In adults, REM sleep is identified by looking at the results of a polysomnography recording (basically, measuring brain waves, heart rate, muscle tone, and the like). With babies, it's not so simple to get a good recording using this method, so researchers use the term "active sleep" to refer to what they believe turns into REM sleep as the baby matures.

- Non-REM or NREM sleep is quiet sleep that is divided into four distinct stages, with each stage producing changes in brain waves, muscle activity, heart function, breathing, and so on. Because

NREM sleep is not fully developed and is difficult to measure in babies, researchers use the term "quiet sleep" to refer to what they believe turns into NREM sleep as the baby matures.

As you sleep, your brain alternates between REM and NREM sleep in cycles that last about 90 minutes. However, the sleep patterns of babies are different from those experienced by older children and adults. Babies' sleep cycles are much shorter, and REM and NREM are distributed differently across the night as compared to adults.

Sleep Patterns for Newborns

Newborns—whose circadian rhythms have not yet developed a day/ night cycle—typically sleep for 2 or 3 hours, wake, feed, and then fall asleep again. They sleep about 16–18 hours a day, with their sleep happening about equally during the day and at night. Newborns don't have a clear distinction between night and day.

Unlike older children and adults, newborns go directly into active (REM) sleep and their sleep is about equally divided between active (REM) and quiet (non-REM) sleep. Researchers speculate that active sleep plays a part in brain development, although they are not sure how.

At about 4 weeks, most babies start sleeping for longer than 2–3 hours at a time at night. They begin to have more active wake periods during the day.

Melissa's Mindset

It's still a great mystery to sleep researchers why young babies have so much active sleep—twice as much as adults. While it's possible that active sleep plays a role in the development of the brain, this has not been proven in humans.

Infant Almanac

Premature infants usually sleep according to their "corrected" age. That is, if your baby was 4 weeks premature, he will sleep like a 2-month-old when he's 3 months old. Be sure to allow preemies extra time to develop sleep patterns before attempting to sleep train them.

Sleep Patterns for Three-Month-Olds

Around this age, the baby begins to sleep for longer periods at one time and for fewer times throughout the day. Most babies also start to sleep more at night. Some babies start skipping one of their nighttime feedings.

At this age, you can start teaching your baby good sleep habits. For example, you can make sure that during the day, she hears daytime noise and is exposed to daylight. You can encourage her to play and stay awake longer. This way she learns that day is different from night. At night, you'll keep her room quiet and dark, and when she wakens, you'll keep your interactions with her low-key.

You can help your baby start to develop good sleep habits now, although you won't do strict sleep training for another 3 months or so.

Sleep Patterns for Six-Month-Olds

By about 6 months, babies no longer go directly to active sleep and the amount of active sleep they get goes down slightly.

Many 6-month-old babies still continue having two—or even more—daytime naps. Six-to-nine-month old babies usually sleep a total of 3–4 hours during the day and 11 or so hours at night. This process of sleeping for longer periods of time is called *sleep consolidation*. The 11-hour nighttime total for babies of this age doesn't always happen in one continuous period.

> **BABY BABBLE**
>
> **Sleep consolidation** is the process during which babies begin sleeping for longer periods of time and not as frequently throughout the day. Another hallmark feature is that they no longer need to feed during the night.

By 6 months, babies' sleep stages have developed enough so that researchers can measure them using polysomnography. So at 6 months, babies' sleep stages are more adult-like and we can begin to use the terms REM and NREM sleep.

The choreography of babies' sleep stages throughout the night is still very different from adults', however. They are still spending more time in REM sleep than adults and will enter into deeper stages of NREM sleep sooner than adults.

Melissa's Mindset

For a yet unknown reason, researchers commonly find a disruption of sleep around 9 months of age and call this a "biobehavioral shift." The shift may be related to the onset of independent locomotion (crawling), separation anxiety, brain development, or a combination of these. It's common for babies who were sleeping very well up to this point to start having problems with going to sleep or with night wakings at around 9 months.

Sleep Patterns for Nine-Month-Olds

An older baby may start having difficulty with separation anxiety—realizing that she is separate from you—and that may cause sleep problems, such as difficulty falling asleep without you or trouble falling asleep after a night waking without your coming in to comfort her.

Infant Almanac

You may be able to comfort your older baby by calling out to him at night instead of being physically present in his room.

Babies this age may also be more easily frightened by noises like barking dogs and thunderstorms, and thus are more likely to have disrupted sleep. They may also be learning to crawl, and this can disrupt sleep.

Sleep Patterns for One-Year-Olds

One-year-olds may continue to have separation anxiety and remain a bit clingy with parents. They may also be able to stand up in their crib but not lie back down—requiring parental intervention at 2 o'clock in the morning.

When a Good Night's Sleep Isn't

You've survived the first few months with your newborn baby—but your newborn is now a 6-month-old baby and still doesn't sleep more than 2 or 3 hours at night.

Of course, all babies continue to have night wakings throughout the first year. It's just that many of them can get themselves to fall back asleep without help from their caregivers.

Or maybe your little one sleeps all right—but getting her to fall asleep in the first place causes untold hours of work and stress.

In such a case, you can use one of the sleep-training approaches described in Parts 2, 3, and 4 to help your baby learn to settle at bedtime or to fall back asleep after a night waking. But sometimes sleep problems indicate something other than poor sleep habits.

If Your Baby Doesn't Sleep Like Other Babies

Many sleep problems—excessive night wakings or difficulty settling for the night—can be helped by using a sleep-training method and by encouraging good sleep habits in your baby. However, your baby's sleep problems may be related to an underlying medical condition, such as seizure disorder, allergies, reflux, ear infections, or teething.

Consult with your pediatrician or disease specialist to help solve sleep problems related to another medical condition. A sleep specialist can also work with you to help solve these problems. See Chapter 19 for more information on sleep training children with special needs.

Melissa's Mindset

There is some new research showing that sleep is disrupted when babies are learning how to walk. Perhaps they're practicing during sleep all night long, as we do when we learn something new (think of when you first learn to ride a bike or type or ski). Regardless of the reason, there is some evidence that sleep becomes disrupted when babies start walking.

Infant Almanac

It's important to keep in mind that your baby's sleep patterns change as she develops. So, if you're a lucky parent who has a young infant who sleeps through the night, it's likely that at some point you will have to deal with disrupted sleep (and mercifully, the opposite is also true).

Melissa's Mindset

Medications used to treat some medical conditions can cause sleep problems in babies and children. Discuss your concerns with your baby's pediatrician or specialist. A change in medication, dosage, or dosing schedule could help.

Infant Almanac

Remember, all babies are different, especially when it comes to sleep/wake cycles. One baby may sleep through the night at 6 weeks while another may be 6 months before this momentous event occurs. Be patient, but don't be afraid to seek help from your pediatrician or a sleep specialist if you're concerned about your baby's sleep.

Unhappy Baby Alert

Babies exposed to secondhand smoke (even prenatally) are more likely to develop apnea.

Some sleep problems are actually due to medical conditions called sleep disorders. These are medical problems that are directly related to sleeping. For example, sleep apnea (cessation of breathing), also called sleep-disordered breathing, can occur in infants and children (and of course adults). Not only can it be a serious medical problem, but it also affects the quality of your child's sleep.

Apnea may be accompanied by fever or other symptoms, or it may be present without other symptoms. A related condition, obstructive apnea, happens when the baby's airway is obstructed (partially blocked), perhaps by congestion, a congenital malformation, or enlarged tonsils or adenoids.

Most apneas clear up and do not cause long-term harm, but apnea may signal a risk for Sudden Infant Death Syndrome (SIDS) or may require resuscitation. For these reasons, you should always consult your pediatrician if you're concerned about apnea. Your pediatrician can recommend strategies for dealing with sleep apnea in your baby or child.

Sleep apnea should not be confused with *periodic breathing*, which is normal in infants.

BABY BABBLE

Periodic breathing is an occasional pause in a baby's breathing that may last up to 10 seconds, related to a newborn's immature respiratory system. It takes a while for breathing responses (and the muscles involved in breathing) to develop in infants. Many parents are alarmed by periodic breathing for fear that it may be sleep apnea. Generally the pause in breathing that babies experience in periodic breathing lasts less than 10 seconds. If it lasts more than 10 seconds, your baby may have apnea. Consult a pediatrician if you're at all concerned.

While central or infant sleep apnea and excessive night wakings are the most common sleep disorder that infants experience, there are others. Consult a pediatrician or sleep specialist if you're concerned.

Melissa's Mindset

Breathing rates in babies are irregular until about 6 months of age. If your baby stops breathing for more than 10 seconds, consider it an emergency and seek help immediately.

Getting Help for Atypical Sleep

Most sleep disruptions in babies are considered "problems" or "disturbances" and can be easily treated using the techniques discussed in this book. In some instances, sleep disruptions are severe and/or caused by an underlying physiological problem. They are then considered "sleep disorders."

It can be difficult to diagnose sleep problems in babies, including sleep disorders such as obstructive apnea.

Melissa's Mindset

Although some clinicians consider excessive night waking in infants a "sleep disorder," others are less comfortable with this diagnosis in infants under 1 year of age, if it does not affect the infant's daytime behavior, and if it is not based on objective measurement of the baby's sleep.

But if you're concerned about your baby's sleep, you may want to seek help. While you may wish to start with your baby's pediatrician, be aware that many pediatricians have very little training in dealing with sleep problems.

You may want to consider bringing your baby to a pediatric sleep specialist, especially if he or she experiences any of the following:

- ◆ Excessive daytime sleepiness
- ◆ Repeated difficulty waking in the morning
- ◆ Excessive night wakings, especially past the age of 1 or 2 years
- ◆ Inconsistency of sleep length
- ◆ Loud or regular snoring

To find a sleep center, check out Appendix B and/or talk with your pediatrician.

The Least You Need to Know

◆ You can help your baby learn to distinguish night from day and to sleep longer at night.

◆ Babies continue to have night wakings throughout their first year (and into their second year and beyond).

◆ Babies' sleep patterns develop over time. Newborns have very different sleep patterns from 1-year-olds.

◆ Occasionally, underlying medical issues or sleep disorders can affect your baby's sleep.

Chapter 3

Sleeping Like a Child

In This Chapter

♦ Understanding how your child's physical, mental, and social maturation can contribute to sleep disruptions throughout his childhood

♦ Knowing when sleep problems may indicate a more serious sleep disorder that may require the intervention of a sleep specialist

♦ Treating underlying medical conditions to help reduce sleep problems

♦ Recognizing typical sleep patterns in children

In this chapter, we'll show you how and why your child's sleep may be disrupted at different stages of life as she grows from toddler to preadolescent (2–12). We'll talk about how to deal with underlying medical conditions to help improve your child's sleep, and we'll cover what you can expect in terms of sleep behavior in your child.

Sleep Disruptions

Even if your baby slept through the night at 6 weeks, the possibility of your child developing sleep problems as he gets older still exists. Owing to mental, emotional, social, and physical changes, your child may develop sleep problems at different stages throughout his life.

As your child matures, you'll find yourself dealing with different causes of sleep problems. However, the sleep-training approaches described in this book can help you handle many of them. See Chapters 16–19 for dealing with specific sleep problems from toddler through preteen years.

Melissa's Mindset

Good sleep habit s can be encouraged through modeling good sleep habits yourself—setting a regular schedule (and keeping it!), practicing a regular bedtime routine, and learning not to rely on crutches (such as sleep aids) to help you sleep.

Even so, establishing good sleep habits early will help you and your child deal with problems down the road and may actually prevent some of them.

For your child, you can encourage good sleep habits by doing the following:

♦ Enforcing consistent bedtimes and wake times, even on weekends and vacations

♦ Creating a comforting bedtime routine

♦ Keeping the child's sleep environment calm, quiet, and dark

♦ Encouraging your child to learn to soothe herself back to sleep if she wakes at night

Physical Changes

As your baby becomes a toddler and then a preschooler, he undergoes many physical changes. His brain develops and organizes a 24-hour sleep cycle. His sleep becomes more adult-like in structure. He goes from being completely helpless to being able to do most of his own self-care. He goes from crying to express everything from pain to fatigue to telling you what he needs and why (sometimes in an annoyingly sarcastic voice).

So it's not surprising that physical changes can lead to changes in sleep habits and to sleep problems. A simple example is the 7-month-old who can stand up in her crib but then can't figure out how to lie back down. So she demands her parents' attention in the middle of the night—whereas even just a few weeks before, she was sleeping through the night (or at least putting herself back to sleep after a night waking).

Another common problem is the older baby who climbs out of her crib. Since this is dangerous, most parents will, at that time, transition their baby to a bed—but now the child can get out of bed at will and seek parental attention. Ignoring a fussy baby suddenly becomes much more difficult, owing to these physical changes.

Emotional Changes

As your baby gets older, she begins to develop a sense of herself as an individual distinct from you. What follows then is often a fierce desire for independence—which includes serious resistance to bedtime. After all, the child thinks you are doing really cool stuff after she goes to bed, and she wants to be part of it.

Unhappy Baby Alert

Your child may also become more anxious and seek more reassurance from you, leading to night wakings that can be extremely disruptive to the entire family.

Mental Changes

Children also develop mentally in ways that can affect sleep. For example, as a child begins to develop independence, he also realizes that he's vulnerable to threats. Younger children, who aren't always able to distinguish fantasy from reality, may then be afraid of ghosts, monsters, or witches. Older children have more realistic fears—they're afraid of natural disasters, "bad guys," and disease.

Common nighttime fears such as these may affect your child's ability

Infant Almanac

Night terrors, nightmares, and sleepwalking are common in children, and are related to mental, emotional, and physical changes that occur in children as they get older. See Chapter 17 for more information on coping with these problems.

to fall asleep. Chapter 17 has specific information on dealing with such fears.

Social Changes

As children mature, they begin to understand that they fit into a social network—family, school, neighborhood. Social challenges and pressures—needing to fit in, feeling slighted by friends—can contribute to a child's level of stress and may make it difficult for her to fall asleep at night. A child who frets about social situations can have difficulty getting enough rest to deal with challenges that come along.

Melissa's Mindset

Bullying is common among school-age children and can cause stress and sleep problems. Bullying should be taken seriously. If you suspect that your child is being bullied, have a talk with him and his teacher. Take steps, such as talking to the school administration, to eliminate the problem.

School problems, such as testing and demanding teachers, also fit in here. Fears of social shortcomings (such as failing to make a friend, being embarrassed by not looking and acting like others, or being more or less advanced academically than others) become more and more common as your child gets older. These problems are very real and should be addressed with compassion and understanding.

What Can You Expect?

Since sleep problems can occur and change over time, be prepared to deal with them as they crop up in your child. Instilling good sleep habits now will help your child in the future.

BABY BABBLE

Sleep deprivation is defined as not getting as much good quality sleep as your body (or your child's body) needs.

Unfortunately, *sleep deprivation* is extremely common in children from preschool on up through the teenage years. Make getting a good night's rest a priority for your child. See Chapter 18 for more information on complications related to sleep deprivation in children.

How Children's Sleep Develops Over Time

All people experience two different kinds of sleep—active REM (rapid eye movement) sleep, during which you dream; and quiet (NREM) sleep, which has four stages characterized by changes in brain waves, muscle movement, eye movement, heart function, breathing, and more. (See Chapter 2 for more information about REM and NREM sleep in babies up to 1 year of age.)

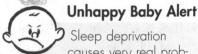

Unhappy Baby Alert

Sleep deprivation causes very real problems for children, including academic difficulties, social problems, and even medical misdiagnosis (for example, mistaking sleep deprivation for Attention Deficit-Hyperactivity Disorder [ADHD]). Being overtired is detrimental to your child's development!

Adults and children over the age of 3 or 4 have similar sleep patterns, going through the 4 stages of NREM sleep:

◆ Stage 1 is the period of transition from drowsiness to sleep and usually lasts only a few minutes.

◆ Stage 2 is a period of light sleep that lasts up to 45 minutes.

◆ Stage 3 is deeper sleep, with slow brain waves and slow, regular breathing.

◆ Stage 4 is the deepest sleep. Stages 3 and 4 may last 60 minutes; then the sleeper returns to Stage 2 sleep.

After one or two cycles of NREM sleep (Stages 1–4), the sleeper usually goes into REM sleep. Most dreams occur during this stage. The first few cycles of REM sleep last only a few minutes, although those periods grow longer as the night progresses.

So, at the beginning of the night, there is a higher proportion of NREM sleep, and by the end of the night, there is a higher proportion of REM sleep. Stages 3 and 4 of NREM sleep are the deepest stages and are considered to be the most restorative. There is some evidence that REM sleep plays an important role in cognitive processing. Both types of sleep are important.

Sleep Patterns for Toddlers

By the time your baby is a toddler, he has probably given up his morning nap but still has an afternoon nap. A good afternoon nap will help him sleep at night, but make sure that the nap doesn't extend too late in the day.

Toddlers sleep about 10–13 hours during every 24-hour period. Often they start climbing out of their cribs at this age, which can cause safety concerns. You may wish to transition your child to a toddler bed, perhaps putting a safety gate across the doorway to prevent late-night escapes. Others suggest keeping your toddler in her crib and putting a crib tent over the top to prevent her from escaping.

Toddlers also resist going to bed at night because they realize that life goes on without them—and they may think they're missing something. Because they're more aware of their dreams, they can feel fearful about sleep time. They may also have trouble sleeping because they're teething, or have medical problems or illnesses.

They can have nightmares, particularly after something frightening has happened to them during the day. They may also have nightmares because of frightening or violent television shows, videos, stories, or video games. Children may not have nightmares immediately after a scary event—sometimes they can occur days or weeks later. Parents are advised to determine the appropriateness of any video, story, game, or show before exposing the child to it in order to prevent unnecessary nightmares. See Chapter 16 for more information.

Melissa's Mindset

With my 4-year-old, the bedtime routine consists of the usual bath or shower, reading stories, brushing teeth, kissing two dogs and the cat, and saying goodnight to Thomas the fish. The routine helps Nickolas to understand that it's bedtime and provides him with comfort because it's the same thing every night.

Sleep Patterns for Preschoolers

Preschoolers are well known for testing limits—including bedtime rules. They will test the limits by requesting one more kiss, one more drink of water, or one more potty break before bed. As we discuss in Chapter 17, it's best to stick to a bedtime routine with this age group and not give in to their attempts to delay bedtime.

Many preschoolers still need an afternoon nap, but even a quiet rest time helps, if your child resists actually sleeping. Usually by age 5 they no longer require this nap. Most need about 10–12 hours of sleep at night. See Chapter 17 for more information.

Sleep Patterns for Gradeschoolers

Some 5-year-olds still need a daytime nap, but most stay awake all day and sleep a little longer at night. Most young children are quite tired after the school day has finished, so quiet evenings and a reasonable bedtime can help keep them from becoming overwrought, cranky, and overtired.

Established bedtime routines are very helpful for children of this age. See Chapter 17 for more information.

> **Infant Almanac**
>
> A study of parents of more than 1,000 school-aged children showed that the most common sleep problem parents encountered was resistance to bedtime.

Sleep Patterns for Older Children

Sleep patterns and circadian rhythms change as people grow older. Adolescents, for example, often prefer staying up later and sleeping later in the morning.

Rather than being simply a social preference, however, research has found that there is a biological shift in the body around puberty that results in adolescents being unable to fall asleep at a "normal" bedtime. This shift in biology makes many adolescents exhibit characteristics of a sleep disorder known as "delayed sleep phase syndrome," in which the body clock tells them to go to bed and wake up much later than is typically acceptable in society, especially with school start times getting progressively earlier as the child matures. More on this in Chapter 18.

> **Infant Almanac**
>
> Studies show that school grades are associated with hours spent sleeping. Students earning As and Bs go to bed earlier and sleep longer than children who have poorer grades.

At around age 11, children need about 10 hours of sleep a day. Teenagers need a little over 9 hours per day. However, most children do not get enough sleep. See Chapter 18 for more information.

Sleep Patterns for Children with Special Needs

Parents of children with special needs often notice sleeping difficulties. For example, children with ADHD are more likely to have night wakings than other children. Premature babies also tend to wake more often at night than full-term infants, especially for the first few months.

Unhappy Baby Alert

Don't forget that medications used to treat medical problems in children with special needs can also disrupt sleep.

Don't dismiss sleep problems in a child with special needs just because you think it's another symptom of the problem. Seeking help can give you and your child a lot of relief.

See Chapter 19 for more information on helping children with special needs get some sleep.

When to Seek Help

If your child has sleep problems that interfere with her ability to settle down for the night or to fall back asleep after a night waking, you may want to try one of the sleep-training approaches described in this book. If the problems are bigger than you can handle on your own, or if you've tried sleep training unsuccessfully, you may want to seek help.

If your child snores, you should also seek help. Snoring is an indication that your child may have obstructive sleep apnea (OSA), the most common sleep disorder in childhood. The bad news is that OSA can cause daytime sleepiness and poor school performance, among other things. The good news is that OSA is treatable. Consult your pediatrician or a pediatric sleep specialist if you have a child who snores loudly and often.

Underlying Medical Conditions

Keep in mind that medical problems such as allergies and asthma may interfere with your child's ability to get a good night's sleep.

Medications used to treat medical conditions may also interfere with sleep. (See Chapter 19 for more information on sleep training children with special needs.) Consult your child's pediatrician or disease specialist for help in overcoming sleep problems associated with such medical conditions.

Common medical ailments that interfere with sleep include ...

- Reflux—when stomach contents come up at least into the esophagus (and sometimes farther) instead of going the other way. It's most common in infancy, but 5–10 percent of children experience symptoms of reflux on a weekly basis. Reflux can interfere with sleep quality, so it's important to consult your pediatrician if it appears to be a problem for your child.

- "Growing pains"— unexplained aches and pains that may keep your child up at night. These are probably from overexertion. A warm bath before bed can help, as can a gentle massage. Encourage your child to take breaks during activity to avoid over-stressing muscles and joints, and encourage a variety of different activities so that no one body part takes all the strain.

- Stomachaches—these may be a stall used at bedtime, or could be related to the flu or another acute illness, or even gas. Stomachaches may be related to stress. If your child complains of stomachaches frequently, have her evaluated by your pediatrician.

> **Melissa's Mindset**
>
> Overweight children are more at risk for sleep apnea, not to mention other medical problems. With your pediatrician, develop a plan to tackle this problem if it affects your child.

- Sleep disorder—your child may suffer from a sleep disorder, such as sleep apnea (see Chapter 2 for more information). These sleep disorders may greatly affect your child's ability to get a good night's sleep. Fortunately, most can be treated effectively. Parasomnias (sleepwalking, sleep talking, sleep terrors, and confusional arousals) are the most common sleep disorders in children after sleep apnea.

Other less common disorders that occur during sleep include:

♦ Restless legs syndrome—a neurologic movement disorder characterized by painful sensations in the legs and an uncontrollable urge to move the legs during sleep.

♦ REM sleep behavior disorder—this disorder occurs more in adults, but has been reported in children. It is characterized by a loss of the usual muscle paralysis during REM sleep so that the person can actually act out dreams.

♦ Sleep paralysis—a condition where the person wakes up and is unable to move, possibly accompanied by hallucinations. This happens when the person wakes up but the body remains paralyzed (as is normal in REM sleep).

♦ Nocturnal eating and drinking syndrome—happens when a child who no longer needs nourishment during the night continues to awaken in order to eat or drink at night.

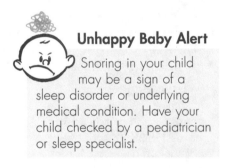

Unhappy Baby Alert

Snoring in your child may be a sign of a sleep disorder or underlying medical condition. Have your child checked by a pediatrician or sleep specialist.

♦ Adjustment sleep disorder—a form of insomnia related to emotional arousal caused by stress (such as starting school or readjusting after a move).

♦ Confusional arousals—very common in children younger than 5; characterized by confusion during and after briefly waking from sleep at the beginning of the night.

Using Medications

If you bring your child to the pediatrician for help with a sleep problem, she may prescribe medications. However, most pediatric sleep specialists see medications as a last resort in treating sleep problems. The following are commonly prescribed medications and what they do.

♦ Antihistamines (yes, we're talking about Benadryl and its cousins): they are highly sedating and can lead babies and children to fall asleep quicker, but there are side effects and they should not be used over the long run. They also don't help children to sleep through the night, just to get to sleep quicker in the first place.

♦ Chloral hydrate: used as a sedative, effective in single dose for medical or dental procedures. There's no evidence that it's safe for repeated use in young children for sleep problems. Using it for sleep problems is highly controversial, and its long-term safety is questioned.

♦ Benzodiazepines (hugely popular, widely prescribed for anxiety, insomnia, etc.): no studies have been done on the effectiveness of these drugs in babies and children, yet they're still prescribed. They suppress deep sleep, so they are useful in treating parasomnias like sleep terrors or sleep walking. They have some pretty major side effects, too: carryover sedation (hangover), cognitive/performance decrements, possible dependence, and relapse once they're discontinued.

♦ Melatonin (hormone, naturally secreted in body during nighttime hours, now synthesized and sold over the counter): supposedly can have a sedative effect. Also used for regulation of sleep-wake schedules. There's no indication that melatonin is safe for young children or that it is effective in typically developing children (no studies have been done). Because it's over-the-counter, the Food and Drug Administration (FDA) does not regulate or test it. Studies that do exist were conducted on populations of children with special needs. The side effects are generally minimal, but one very small study of six children found that four out the six experienced increases in seizures.

Melissa's Mindset

Sleep experts generally discourage the use of sedatives or any of these medications in children. Using sleep-training techniques and treating underlying medical conditions is the preferred course of action.

The Least You Need to Know

♦ Your child's sleep may be disrupted by social, emotional, mental, and physical changes.

◆ Underlying medical problems, such as allergies or asthma, can affect your child's sleep, as can sleep disorders such as apnea.

◆ Instilling good sleep habits in your child now can prevent problems down the road.

◆ Sleep difficulties negatively impact school performance and can worsen or even cause emotional difficulties, such as depression.

Chapter 4

Getting Started

In This Chapter

- ◆ Developing good sleep habits in your baby
- ◆ Choosing the best sleep-training methods for you and your baby or child
- ◆ Exploring myths and misconceptions about sleep
- ◆ Understanding how to adapt sleep-training approaches for your older child

Now what? You've got the baby (or the child) and you're ready to start getting some sleep.

In this chapter, we'll show you what your next steps should be. We'll describe how to match you and your baby to an appropriate sleep-training method, and we'll explain some myths and misconceptions about sleep.

We'll also show you how you can use the methods for older children, with a little bit of tweaking. And we'll let you know when it might *not* be a good idea to sleep train your child.

Discovering Your Parenting and Sleep-Training Philosophy

In Chapter 1, we discussed setting your sleep-training goals—in other words, identifying the sleep problem you're trying to solve. Once you know what you're trying to do, you can move on to figuring out the best way to do it.

Essentially, sleep problems fall into two categories: difficulty settling for the night and difficulty falling back to sleep after night waking.

Melissa's Mindset

You and your partner—and other adults in the household—should be on the same page no matter what sleep-training method you're planning to try. Educate yourself and present your case to the other dealmakers or deal-breakers in the house. Agree together on the approach that is the most likely fit for all of you.

Some babies and children have both problems. If yours is one who has both, you'll want to decide if you want to tackle both problems at once or work on them one at a time.

But that still leaves you with the most important decision you'll make: which sleep-training approach is best for you and your baby?

This is a very individual choice and depends on your parenting philosophy, your personality, and your baby's temperament.

In Chapter 1, we described general differences in the sleep-training approaches. By reading Parts 2 and 3 (Chapters 6 through 15) you'll understand how the different approaches work and what types of parents tend to pick what types of approaches.

You may have a strong feeling that one method will work better for you than another. Follow your instincts! If you feel strongly that attachment parenting is your philosophy and that a family-bed approach (Chapter 12) is the right solution for you and your child, then you owe it to yourself to at least give it a try.

But what if you don't feel strongly about one particular method over another?

Melissa's Mindset

Although I knew the type of parent I was and the type of child I had from the start, I still tried to let Nickolas "cry it out" at one point during the first year of his life. My "cry it out" attempt lasted 10 minutes one night and I never went back. Some parents and babies just aren't cut out for this technique, just as some parents and babies aren't cut out for the less rigid techniques. Rest assured that you and your baby can get a good night's sleep once you find a technique that works for everyone.

Then you need to take stock of your parenting philosophy, your personality, your habits, your child's personality, and your ability to withstand a crying baby. If you know you'll wimp out at the first whimper from your baby, then the "ignore it" approach (Chapter 6) is not going to work for you.

On the other hand, maybe you're a highly scheduled adult, dependent on a daily routine. A laissez-faire "he'll outgrow it" approach may reduce *you* to tears.

In other words, be honest with yourself and about yourself. If your child has night wakings, can you discipline yourself to set the alarm two or three or four times a night to wake so that you can, in turn, wake your baby before she starts to cry ("scheduled awakenings" approach, Chapter 10)? If you just can't imagine doing this, then try another approach first.

Melissa's Mindset

I don't recommend trying one sleep-training approach after another. Sometimes at the first challenge, a parent will give up the method. Unfortunately, this can communicate the wrong message to your baby or child and could actually be more harmful than not bothering with a sleep-training method at all. This is why it's important to choose wisely!

Matching the Method to Your Baby

While your parenting philosophy and your own personality are important factors to consider when choosing a sleep-training approach, don't forget the most important consideration of all: your child.

All children are different and they respond differently to the various sleep-training approaches. Even in one family, different children respond to different methods differently. So what worked for your older child may not be effective (or as effective) with your second child.

Melissa's Mindset

Even Dr. Ferber, famed for the method of sleep training called "graduated extinction" (or "ignore but check"—see Chapter 7), now says in the newly revised version of this book that this technique may not be helpful to particularly anxious children. It's best to choose a technique based on the fit between your parenting philosophy and your child's personality.

Before making your decision, consider what you know about your child's personality. A particularly clingy, anxious child may have increased anxiety if you use an "ignore" method with him (see Chapter 6) but may respond better to an "ignore but check" method (Chapter 7) where he's reassured that you're there and will check on him occasionally or to an approach that does not involve tears (see Part 3). The "ignore it but be there" approach, alternatively, may simply reinforce his clinginess (see Chapter 8).

By the same token, a fairly easy-going baby without serious sleep problems could probably do just fine if you use the "wait it out" approach (Chapter 14) for those mild problems or occasional disturbances she does experience.

When Your Sleep-Training Method Isn't Working

When you embark on any sleep-training approach, it's important for you to understand how it works, to be prepared for challenges, and to commit to seeing it through.

But what happens when a given method simply isn't working for you? And when do you know it isn't?

Chucking one method and trying another requires some careful evaluation. In each of the method chapters (Parts 2 and 3) we give an estimate of how long it will take for the method to work. Allowing a little leeway for error, if you've tried for longer than the given range, it may be time to rethink your strategy. Follow these guidelines:

◆ First, you'll want to honestly ask yourself if you've been using the approach as described. Was your Ferberizing (Chapter 7) interrupted by a weeklong visit with Grandma and Grandpa? If so, then maybe keeping at it a little longer will work.

◆ Next, if you have used the approach as recommended, you may simply need to tweak it for it to be a success. See Chapter 15 on how to combine strategies to increase your likelihood of success with a given method.

◆ Finally, if you've tried the method as recommended for at least as long as suggested, but it's not working and you don't feel as if you can continue trying the method, then it's time to go ahead and make a change.

◆ If you do decide that your method isn't working, don't just try the next approach on the list and hope it works out. Try to understand why the method you originally chose didn't work for you. This will help you choose a more effective method to try next.

If you have decided on a technique and feel comfortable with it, then it's extremely important to see it through, especially if you have decided to try one of the "ignore" approaches. Once you have made the decision to try ignoring, it's essential that you follow the approach and stick with it. If you try it on night one and then decide you can't handle it on night two, then try it again on night three, you have already made the problem worse by being inconsistent.

> **Infant Almanac**
>
> If you can't stick with a given method because it's harder than you anticipated it would be—for example, if you simply can't listen to your baby cry for more than 3 minutes—then go ahead and stop, evaluate what worked for you and what didn't, and try again with another method that you're more likely to follow successfully.

Of course, if on night two you realize that this is not the approach for you, then go ahead and stop. However, you need to know that if you change your mind, it will take longer to achieve success. Once you've been inconsistent, your child will take longer to respond to your sleep-training efforts.

> **Infant Almanac**
>
> Reactive choices occur when you react to a challenge without planning for it. For example, you soothe your baby to sleep every night by driving all over town because you don't have a better approach mapped out. Proactive choices occur when you decide how you're going to respond to a given sleep problem and then follow through on your plan. Reactive choices can actually cause or worsen sleep problems, whereas proactive approaches are less likely to cause difficulties.

Promoting Good Sleep Early On

Although you can't sleep train a very young baby, you can promote and encourage good *sleep habits* from the beginning. Even if you don't follow a sleep-training method, you can help your baby (or child) develop good sleep habits just by using these techniques:

- Be a good role model.

- Keep a regular bedtime and wake time schedule—for you and your child.

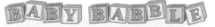

Sleep habits are routines and rituals that affect how you fall asleep and how well you sleep.

- Keep the hours around bedtime calm and stress-free.

- Keep the child's sleeping environment calm, dark, and quiet.

- Make sleep a priority for everyone in the family.

When Sleep Training Is a Bad Idea

While encouraging good sleep habits in your child is always helpful, there may be certain times when sleep training your child is a bad idea.

For example, if your child is ill, especially with something more serious than a cold, now is not the time to start Ferberizing her. If you're dealing with medical problems, you may choose to delay the additional stress of sleep training until after the treatment is concluded or your child is more stable and you've developed a more settled daily routine.

For the same reason, you may wish to put off sleep training with a child who is dealing with trauma or other mental or emotional issues.

This is not to say you shouldn't encourage a good night's rest—you should. Sleep deprivation can certainly worsen mental, emotional, and physical challenges. However, it may make sense for you to conserve your energy to solve the big, immediate problems and then work on sleep training.

You can also expect some setbacks with your child's sleep during the following common situations:

Melissa's Mindset

Even something as simple as a cold can disrupt sleep patterns, so trying to change things when your baby is sick is never a good idea. In fact, if you have gone through sleep training with a child and then the child gets sick, he may regress and you may need to retrain following the illness.

Unhappy Baby Alert

It's not a good idea to start sleep training if you have a trip planned within the next few weeks or if you'll have visitors and expect that the baby's schedule will be disrupted during their visit. Be sure that you have a good amount of time at home before trying anything new.

- Your child has a serious physical, mental, emotional, or social challenge.

- A close friend or family member (or pet) is ill or injured.

- A close friend or family member (or pet) has died.

- You and your partner, close friends, or relatives separate or divorce.

- You move from one location to another, even if it's just across town.

- Your family experiences an emotional upheaval such as a job loss.

In any of these cases, reassuring your child about his fears and encouraging good sleep can help, although you may want to put off sleep training (especially the stricter "ignore" approaches) at least until the immediate crisis has passed.

Myths and Misconceptions About Sleep

As you try to get your child to learn good sleep habits, you'll probably hear lots of well-intentioned advice from other parents, some of which is helpful and some of which is plain wrong.

Feeding the Baby Solids Helps Promote Sleep

If your 3- or 4-month-old still wakes up hungry during the night, Grandma might suggest feeding solid foods (such as cereal) in the evening to help the baby sleep. Babies used to be fed solids earlier than is recommended now.

Melissa's Mindset

When looking through a friend's old baby things, I came across a note from the doctor in the late 1960s recommending cereal when the baby was 4 weeks old! Our understanding of what works with babies and children continually evolves.

However, there's no relationship between starting solid food and sleeping through the night. Starting a baby on solids too early may lead to a greater risk of the baby developing food allergies later. The American Academy of Pediatrics recommends exclusive breastfeeding for the first 4 to 6 months of life, followed by a gradual introduction of solids.

Napping Interferes with Nighttime Rest

All babies and young children need naps. By the time most children are toddlers, they're down to one nap, in the afternoon. By about age 5, most children have outgrown this nap. But having a nap, especially after a less-than-ideal night's sleep, won't interfere with your child's nighttime sleep unless the nap occurs too close to bedtime. In fact, paradoxically, a well-rested baby tends to sleep better at night. Often, if children are overtired, they sleep worse at night.

In other words, napping is routine and necessary in young children. If your preschooler's nap does seem to interfere with her sleeping at night, try moving the start time so that the nap is over by 3 P.M. This will help ensure that your child is reasonably sleepy at bedtime.

Sleep Patterns Are Hereditary

All children develop certain sleep patterns, and although some part of the pattern is genetic, it isn't necessarily hereditary and it is certainly strongly influenced by environment, experience, and training.

So just because you're a night owl, it doesn't mean your baby will be one, too. But because you're a night owl, you might model night-owl behaviors and, without meaning to, encourage your little one to become a night owl, too.

Some sleep disorders, such as narcolepsy, are thought to be hereditary. So if the baby's biological parents have a sleep disorder such as narcolepsy, you should let your doctor know this and keep an eye out for symptoms in your child.

Bigger Babies Sleep Better

The idea that a larger baby sleeps better than a smaller one is simply not true. There's no correlation between a baby's weight and the quality of his sleep.

A premature baby, however, will sleep according to his "corrected" age. So a baby who was born 6 weeks premature will sleep more like a 6-week-old when he's 3 months old.

Gifted Babies Sleep Less

Some parents believe that gifted babies sleep less than their "average" peers. But there is no correlation between a child's cognitive development and the quality of her sleep. So if your child sleeps soundly, rest assured that she just might be gifted!

A Later Bedtime Equals a Later Waketime

If you've ever tried this, you know it simply isn't true. Although it seems like common sense that a baby who sleeps, say, 10 hours at night will sleep those 10 hours no matter when you put him down, that's not actually the case.

Just as we are programmed to wake up at a certain time every day, babies are, too, and it's much less likely that they will hit the snooze button and go back to sleep. To boot, you'll have an overtired, miserable, sleep-deprived child to deal with all day. Trust us: don't try this at home.

Adapting the Methods for Older Kids

You're never too old for sleep training—and neither is your child. Everyone can benefit from improved sleep habits because the effects of sleep deprivation are so serious.

Of course, it's easiest to start sleep training when your child is young—preferably a baby around 6 months of age. At this age, you can teach her to self-soothe; she's capable of sleeping for longer chunks of time; and she's not yet old enough to climb out of bed every 7 seconds to ask for just one more drink or another visit to the potty.

But if you missed that window of opportunity, never fear: you can sleep train an older child, though you will encounter different challenges.

See Chapters 16–19 for more about sleep training children from toddler to preteen.

Getting Your Older Child to Cooperate

Getting a toddler to stop resisting bedtime is different from getting your 12-year-old to back away from the computer and get to bed.

Firmness, consistency, and commitment make all the difference. If you let your 2-year-old get out of bed sometimes when he cries but not at other times, you're actually creating more of a monster than you would if you let him get out of bed every time he cries. That's because intermittent reinforcement (rewarding a behavior only sometimes) is the most powerful way to ensure that a behavior continues.

Getting your older child's buy-in might include discussing the effect of sleep deprivation in ways that matter to her. For example, you might explain to an 8-year-old that not getting enough sleep means she's more likely to argue with her friends (increased irritability) or hurt herself when she's playing (lack of focus). An older child might be more concerned if you explain the correlation between poor sleep and poor grades.

Your older child can also help create a sleep plan. He may be able to brainstorm ideas that would help him develop better sleep habits. Perhaps he could socialize before dinner instead of just before bed. Or perhaps he could do his homework right after coming home from school instead of after dinner. Or perhaps he could reduce the number of activities he's involved in, meaning he has more downtime, time to relax, and time to play on the computer and socialize with friends.

Matching the Method to Your Older Child

Just as you match the sleep-training method to your baby, you want to match the method to your older child.

The "ignore" method (Chapter 6) may have worked when your baby was 6 months old, but now that she's a 10-year-old, she might find it insulting, not to mention that it just won't work. You can lead a pre-teen to bed, but you can't make her sleep.

Take your child's personality into consideration as you choose the right approach to try.

The Least You Need to Know

- ◆ The sleep-training approach you use will depend on your parenting philosophy, your personality, and your baby's temperament.

- ◆ Sometimes a given method simply doesn't work with your child. In that case, you'll need to try an alternative approach.

- ◆ When your child is experiencing mental, emotional, physical, or social changes, you may want to delay sleep training.

- ◆ You can avoid sleep-training missteps by being aware of common sleep myths and misconceptions.

Chapter 5

Pampering Parents

In This Chapter

- ◆ Why taking care of yourself helps you take care of your baby
- ◆ Finding ways to get some sleep
- ◆ Seeking help when you need it
- ◆ Working out a system with your partner so all people involved get what they need

"Pampering yourself" and "new baby" don't exactly go together. We know! But take it from us—paying attention to your own needs will make you a better, more relaxed parent and may help everyone in your family maintain good relationships with each other.

In this chapter, we'll offer some suggestions for taking care of yourself while also taking care of your baby.

Getting Some Sleep Yourself

Adults need about 8 hours of sleep each night, although this can range from 7–10 hours. People who get less than 7 hours per night are generally sleep deprived—they get drowsy during the day, become more irritable, have difficulty focusing, and suffer other problems.

Sleep deprivation makes it hard to be a good parent, so the greater the emphasis you place on getting enough sleep, the more effective you're likely to be as a parent. But when your baby isn't sleeping through the night, *you're* not sleeping through the night.

Unhappy Baby Alert

Many new parents try to keep up with their lives just as they did before baby was born. This is a recipe for sleep deprivation! For at least the first few weeks, it's okay to order take-out, eat off paper plates, leave the vacuum cleaner in the closet, and have someone else do the laundry!

So what can you do? For the first few weeks, follow your baby's lead—at least when it comes to sleep (crying is optional). Sleep when your baby does—even if it's in the middle of *Desperate Housewives*. (This is where learning how to program that VCR or DVR can come in handy.)

Dealing with Medical Problems

Medical problems, including depression and anxiety, can affect your ability to get some sleep. Make sure you get treatment so that you can enjoy your new baby and parent him the best you can. And don't forget that adults can have sleep disorders such as sleep apnea, too. Be sure to seek treatment for your sleep problems.

Some degree of the blues following pregnancy is common. This can range from *baby blues* to *postpartum depression* to *postpartum psychosis*.

BABY BABBLE

Baby blues are generally mild feelings of sadness, mood swings, or periods of crying that go away in a couple of weeks following birth.

Postpartum depression is a severe, longer-lasting depression.

Postpartum psychosis is an extreme but rare form of depression involving hallucinations and delusions.

Inadequate sleep can make the depression worse, and in some cases, the depression itself can cause sleep problems over and above what you experience from the baby's waking.

Either way, it's important to take care of yourself. If you have feelings of sadness, lack of energy, trouble concentrating, and feelings of worthlessness that are debilitating and last for more than a couple of weeks, you should talk to your doctor and seek treatment. This is the most important thing you can do for you and your baby.

Melissa's Mindset

Don't forget that medications you're taking for medical problems may create sleep problems. Consult your physician—you may be able to switch to a medication that won't interfere with your sleep.

Creating Your Own Good Sleep Habits

You'll want to make sure that you're following good sleep habits, especially after the first few weeks when your topsy-turvy life settles down a bit.

Here are some tactics for helping ensure a good night's sleep:

◆ Keep a regular schedule.

◆ Avoid caffeine and other stimulants, especially near bedtime.

◆ Avoid smoking and being around smoke.

◆ Skip the after-dinner drink— alcohol disrupts sleep.

◆ Sleeping pills and sedatives don't solve sleep problems in the long term—make real lifestyle changes instead.

◆ Exercise—not too close to bedtime—can help you sleep.

◆ A light snack may help you drift off to dream land.

Melissa's Mindset

If you've had sleep problems throughout your adult life, it may be worth it to seek a consultation with a sleep specialist. Now that you're a parent, you need to be well rested—not to mention the importance of being a good role model for your child when it comes to sleep. Taking this step can help not just you but your whole family.

◆ A regular bedtime routine for yourself—including wind-down time—can help you sleep better.

◆ Relax about everything that isn't getting done.

◆ Make sleep a priority—plan for it.

Creating a Good Sleep Environment

You'll also want to make sure your sleep environment is conducive to sleeping. Just as you want to keep your child's room cool, dark, and quiet, do the same for your own room. Try the following:

◆ Indulge in a comfortable pillow, mattress, and bedding.

◆ Use a fan or white-noise machine to mask street noise.

◆ Move the television and computer out of the bedroom.

◆ Don't eat, read, or talk on the phone in bed.

◆ Use your bedroom only for sleep and, well, you know. Don't put your home office next to your bed or you'll be thinking about all the work you haven't finished when you should actually be sleeping.

◆ The smell of lavender is restful, so use lavender sachet, potpourri, or air freshener.

You should feel relaxed when you walk into your bedroom, so make it a habit to keep it clear of clutter—hang up clothes or put them in the hamper; throw a comforter on the bed to "make" it.

Managing Your Expectations

Understanding what to expect of your baby—and yourself—can help you get through the most difficult sleep challenges. For example, knowing that it could be months before your baby sleeps through the night may convince you that you need to change your schedule in order to get some shuteye.

As your child gets older, sticking with clear expectations can help everyone get some sleep. Keep up good sleep habits and make bedtime firm and non-negotiable.

Manage expectations of yourself, too. Can you really be supermom, a devoted trial attorney, and breastfeed your triplets on demand? Maybe getting a little help and letting go of some of your expectations would help you get some sleep.

Melissa's Mindset

Even after your baby is sleeping through the night, you may find that you're still waking in the middle of the night. That's to be expected—it will just take a little time for your sleep patterns to return to normal.

Because you have demands on your time even when you've been up all night with a wakeful baby, you have to ask yourself if you really need to do what you think you have to do. Learning to just say no can make all the difference sometimes. Having a child means setting limits on other demands so that you can be a calm and sane parent. If you have to choose between getting some sleep and dusting the furniture, you know what we're going to tell you to do!

Melissa's Mindset

Keeping a sense of humor about your situation can sometimes help you get through the tough sleep trials. Try not to take everything too seriously.

Tag-Team Parenting

One of the best ways you can help yourself is to learn to ask for help. Mothers especially try to do it all themselves, but this is not in your best interest—or your child's.

Fathers are sometimes reluctant to jump in and take care of business since Mom seems to be handling everything. If this is the case for you, sit down together and spell out what Dad can and should do. Both partners should contribute, although their contributions may be different. When baby is tough to soothe, maybe Mom can hand her off to Dad for a gentle massage. (See Chapter 21 for more information on infant and child massage.)

Develop a tag-team parenting approach so that no one is overly burdened with nighttime baby duty. Trade off nights, if possible. If Mom is still breastfeeding, at least Dad can get the baby from her crib and bring her to bed.

When you're stressed and agitated, your baby can sense it, which may lead to fussiness. Turning over the baby to a fresh caretaker when you're exhausted is best for everyone. One approach that many parents find helpful is for each partner to develop an activity or hobby (maybe just seeing a movie with friends) that they do by themselves. Knowing that every Monday night you're off kid patrol and can do whatever you want makes a big difference the rest of the week. Your partner can have Wednesdays off. You'll be surprised at how a brief break like this will help you feel energized and ready to deal.

> **Infant Almanac**
>
> In addition to having some solo time, many partners find that they have to work hard to carve out time together. Find a trusted sitter and make a date night once a week or so—even if it's just to go to the grocery store.

If you don't have a partner, you will definitely need extra help. Enlist a grandmother, a sibling, or even a trusted neighborhood teen to give you some time off. Jennifer used to hire a sitter just so she could take a nap! Just spending an hour over coffee with friends can recharge you. Or hire a cleaning service so you can get to bed at a reasonable hour. Many communities have inexpensive respite-care organizations just waiting for your call. There's no right or wrong way to use help. Ask for help and you'll definitely be a calmer, saner parent. Being healthy and well rested is the best gift you can give your child, so make it a priority!

Staying the Course

You're in this for the long haul, so you should plan for that instead of reacting to a given problem when it happens. This means planning for help so that you're not frantically trying to find it at the last minute. Even before your baby is born you can investigate community resources, find out who your friends use for babysitting, visit daycare centers, and the like.

Develop coping strategies for dealing with your child's sleep challenges. For example, you may find that learning certain relaxation methods can help you stay calm despite your baby's repeated night wakings.

Such relaxation methods may include learning to meditate, or taking a warm bath at night. It might be practicing Tai Chi first thing in the morning, before baby awakens. Or it might be having one night out per week with your friends. Or some combination of the above. Discover strategies that work for you—and use them!

 Melissa's Mindset

One of the best resources to find knowledgeable people to help care for your child is your local community college or university. Check to see if they have a child-development program and, if so, try recruiting potential helpers by putting up a flyer or announcing your position on a listserv.

The Least You Need to Know

◆ You should make getting sleep a priority for you.

◆ Asking for help is good for you and your baby.

◆ Planning how you and your partner will cope with your baby's or child's sleep challenges can reduce problems.

◆ Developing relaxation strategies can help you cope.

Part 2

Crying It Out

"Extinction" methods of sleep training are based on the idea that ignoring your baby's tears is sometimes the best way to teach him how to fall asleep—and to fall back to sleep when he wakes up.

In this part, we'll cover the "cry it out" sleep-training approaches—and yes, there are several, some of which are less abrupt than others.

Chapter 6

I Can't Hear You ...

In This Chapter

- The "ignore it" sleep-training approach
- Being proactive rather than reactive with your baby
- Developing a schedule for you and your baby
- Learning to let your baby cry herself to sleep without inter-fcring

Were all those people who said, "Your life will never be the same after you have a baby" wrong? Maybe so! In this chapter, we're going to show you strategies for living your life pretty much the way you always did, despite the bald-headed, fist-waving charmer you're welcoming to the fold.

You can use these strategies to help your new baby fit into your schedule—instead of changing your schedule to fit the baby. If knowing what's going to happen all day, every day, is important to you, you'll find the answers to how to get your baby on board in this chapter. We'll explain how the "ignore it" approach creates a reliable routine for sleeptime. We'll also describe how you can solve sleep problems in your older baby by letting him cry it out.

The "Ignore It" Approach

You're a parent, not a peer. So you're responsible for teaching your baby how to have self-control (and other virtues). That's the foundation of the "ignore it" approach. Of course, the "ignore it" approach isn't quite as simple as, well, ignoring it.

Researchers refer to it as the "ignoring/systematic extinction" approach, and it focuses on teaching your child how to fall asleep without your help. Not surprising, then, that one of the main features of the approach is ignoring your baby when she cries at bedtime. But first you must lay the right foundation during the day—by establishing a 3-hour schedule of feeding your baby and then keeping her awake before allowing her to nap again.

What It Is

In the "ignore it" approach, you establish that you're in charge of your baby, not the other way around.

- ◆ Start by creating a feeding and sleeping schedule for your baby early in his infancy.

- ◆ Once your baby is older (four to six months), begin ignoring his crying at naptime and at nighttime when you put him down to sleep.

- ◆ According to this theory, ignoring the cries will eventually teach your baby to soothe himself to fall asleep at bedtime and after night wakings.

Creating a Routine

In the "ignore it" approach, your baby learns to adjust to you instead of you adjusting to your baby. You fit your child into your schedule instead of the other way around.

The "ignore it" approach is not just a method of sleep training, but a method of directing and controlling your new baby's entire eating time-waketime-sleep time schedule. According to one of the most popular supporters of this approach, Gary Ezzo, the cycle should go like this:

> **Infant Almanac**
>
> The "ignore it" method is the opposite of the "child-centered" approach to parenting (see Chapter 12), which is thought to be destructive to the family and to encourage self-centeredness in the child.

◆ Eating time—you wake the child (or he may wake naturally) and offer a feeding.

◆ Wake time—after feeding, you have a period of play time with your baby, keeping him awake for awhile and giving him attention.

◆ Nap time—after waketime/playtime is over, you put your baby back down to sleep.

According to Ezzo, from the time you bring your baby home from the hospital, your goal is to establish this sequence. Since babies can't regulate their own sleep and eating habits, the parents must do it for them. The "ignore it" approach means working toward having approximately the same amount of time pass from one feeding/waking/sleeping cycle to the next. However, it may be difficult to impose such a schedule on a newborn.

Some supporters of this approach are more flexible, emphasizing the need to watch the baby's signals and to put the baby to bed when he looks drowsy. In other words, you can let the baby sleep no matter how much (or little) time has passed since the last nap. This more flexible variation is less parent-driven, but does require a strict bedtime routine—the baby goes to bed at the same time every night.

> **Melissa's Mindset**
>
> No research-based evidence shows that erratic schedules keep the baby's brain from organizing sleep and wake cycles. As discussed in Chapter 2, babies develop day-night rhythms in sleep and wakefulness by living in a world where darkness and lightness alternate regularly.

Creating a predictable schedule means that you know what to expect and can plan the day's events more easily than if you simply react to the baby's demands. Erratic schedules, believe supporters of this approach, prevent your baby's brain from organizing her sleep and wake cycles.

Sticking to a Schedule

The "ignore it" approach requires using a very specific daily schedule with your child. Ezzo calls this "parent-directed feeding" because he believes that your feeding philosophy determines whether your baby *sleeps through the night* (which usually happens between the ages of 7 and 9 weeks, according to Ezzo).

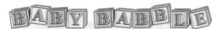

People define **sleeping through the night** in different ways. Some consider midnight to 5 A.M. as sleeping through. This is important for parents to keep in mind when considering the claims made by supporters of different sleep-training approaches.

Parent-directed feeding requires the parent to consider hunger cues (the baby crying), plus clock time (how long it has been since the last feeding), plus parental assessment (is the baby crying for some other reason—a wet diaper, an annoying sibling?) to determine whether it is feeding time.

Other supporters of this approach agree that establishing a routine eating and sleeping schedule helps you and your baby thrive.

Routine feeding creates routine hunger so the baby will become hungry at predictable times, according to "ignore it" gurus. The whole cycle of eating, waking, and sleeping can be conducted according to a schedule.

And in This Corner: Supporters of This Approach

The most popular book about this approach is *On Becoming Babywise* by Gary Ezzo and Robert Bucknam, M.D. They reached their conclusions about parent-directed feedings and other features of the "ignore it" approach from conducting a small unpublished study of 520 infants and from anecdotal evidence based on their experiences (Ezzo is a parent educator and Bucknam is a pediatrician). Their book has been widely read and has found many supporters among parents and pediatricians.

Marc Weissbluth, M.D., a well-known and well-respected pediatrician and sleep researcher, advocates a more flexible version of the "ignore it" approach while emphasizing the importance of schedules in *Healthy Sleep Habits, Happy Child.*

Using This Approach

Following the "ignore it" approach requires avoiding so-called child-centered pitfalls. Parents should focus on ...

♦ Life continuing as it always has.

♦ Maintaining relationships with spouse, family, and friends, with and without the child being present.

♦ Developing a consistent eat-waketime-sleep schedule with the baby.

Avoiding Sleep Props

When it's bedtime, you put the baby to bed without using "props"—activities or objects intended to soothe the baby and lull her to sleep. Examples of sleep props that are thought to interfere with sleep training are the following:

♦ Nursing the baby to sleep

♦ Rocking the baby to sleep

♦ Sleeping with the baby

Ask your friends about the desperate measures they've used to get the baby to sleep—the rocking chair is just the start. Soon you'll be driving all over town because the motion of the car soothes the baby to sleep. But don't stop—the baby will wake up if you do!

That's the reason supporters of this approach are so vehement about *not* using props. They feel that babies

Melissa's Mindset

Research shows that most babies don't sleep through the night at 9 weeks, especially breast-fed babies. Most babies continue to wake at night through the first year of life, but some babies can put themselves back to sleep—enabling *parents* to sleep through the night.

can naturally learn to fall asleep on their own without props, and that if you use props, you will interfere with this process and also create work, anxiety, and frustration for yourself.

Instead of using a prop or waiting for your baby to fall asleep before putting her to bed, put your baby to bed while she is awake. Then your baby will learn to fall asleep without outside help.

If directed by parents, typical infants will sleep through the night by 9 weeks, according to Ezzo.

Step-by-Step

Parents begin by enforcing the eat-waketime-sleep schedule with their infant. They may use parent-directed feeding, previously described, to determine when it is time to feed the baby.

Infant Almanac

Usually the last 1 to 1½ hours of the 3-hour cycle should be spent sleeping, with the remaining 1½ to 2 hours divided between feeding and playing. Babies who are slower feeders may have a shorter playtime before they go back to sleep.

Melissa's Mindset

Many sleep experts, including those who disagree with the "ignore it" approach and those who agree with it, recommend that parents not let their children cry it out until the baby is older. Most agree that it is inappropriate for infants younger than 4 to 6 months of age to cry themselves to sleep.

Using this approach from the beginning means that you'll be trying to keep your newborn awake for a little while after each feeding (except for the middle-of-the-night feedings). Remember the cycle: eat-waketime-sleep. The schedule must be established from the beginning.

At the newborn stage, the goal is to establish an eat-waketime-sleep schedule that recurs every 3 hours or so, from the beginning of one feeding to the next. To prevent the baby from falling asleep while eating, which means the baby doesn't get enough to eat in order to sleep for the longer periods of time needed for this approach to work, you might tickle him, change his clothes, or play a little.

If the child sleeps longer than the 3-hour cycle permits, you should wake him up. While this may sound counter-productive, it actually helps to establish the cycle, according to Ezzo. Other supporters of the approach, such as Weissbluth, disagree and encourage babies to sleep through the day. A well-rested baby is more likely to sleep well at night, they believe.

Ignore the Crying

Now we come to the "ignore it" part of the "ignore-it" method. Although some supporters of the "ignore it"

> **Melissa's Mindset**
>
> Waking the baby at the end of the 3-hour cycle helps to establish the parent-imposed cycle, not the child's sleep-wake rhythm. There is no research to show that the sleep-wake rhythm is facilitated by an imposed schedule. Instead try allowing the baby to sleep when she seems tired, exposing the baby to sunlight during the day, and keeping lights off at night.

approach disagree, most sleep researchers say that if you use the "ignore it" approach, you should not start ignoring the baby's cries at bedtime until the baby is 4 to 6 months old.

When you're establishing the schedule, start with a consistent first feeding time and a consistent bedtime each night. This will allow for all days to follow a similar routine. According to Ezzo, by the time the baby is 8 or 9 weeks old and can sleep through the night, your job, once you've put the baby to bed for the night, is to ignore any crying. However, most experts agree that actually ignoring your baby's cries shouldn't start until your baby is 4 to 6 months old. Of course it's easier to say "ignore it" than to do it!

Supporters of this method emphasize that you need to let the baby cry it out consistently. If you go back and forth between ignoring the baby and soothing the baby, you merely reinforce the idea that you'll sometimes appear if the baby cries—which encourages the baby to cry even more.

Disruptions to the Schedule

Occasionally your baby's schedule will be disrupted through travel, visiting relatives, and similar situations. Supporters of the "ignore it" approach say that you should take these special circumstances into consideration. For example, if it's not "time" to feed the baby, but the baby is fussy and you're on a flight home for Thanksgiving, consider the other people's feelings and feed the child instead of sticking firmly to the schedule. Everyone aboard will thank you.

As soon as the disruption is over, however, you need to go back to the schedule and the "ignore it" system. That means getting back on schedule as soon as possible and going "cold turkey" again with sleep times. After a disruption, the baby is likely to cry more than usual, but supporters of this approach say that's to be expected and you should ignore it.

Some supporters of the "ignore it" approach, such as Weissbluth, say that bedtime should be firm no matter what the circumstances. An overtired child is difficult to get to sleep.

Challenges You'll Encounter

Sticking to the routine is key. When it is bedtime, the baby goes down. Your ability to ignore the crying without bursting into sobs yourself will be the biggest challenge you face. Ignore the fussing and crying that will occur. Usually the crying period lasts no more than about 20 minutes. Supporters of this approach point out that crying is natural and that trying to stop it may actually increase stress rather than decrease it.

According to Weissbluth, this "cold turkey" approach is more effective and less stressful than other more gradual approaches (such as the "ignore but check" method described in Chapter 7). He says that starting early with this type of training reduces bouts of crying. He also emphasizes the importance of consistency with the sleep-training method. Going back and forth between permissiveness and firmness creates problems.

Unhappy Baby Alert

Of course, sometimes crying is not normal or typical and you should not just ignore it. For example, a sharp cry of pain is something you should check. A cry that sounds different from the normal falling-asleep cry should also be checked.

If the baby wakes up too early from a nap, don't immediately pick her up. Your baby may settle back down again to finish the nap, but won't do so if you intervene. Babies who frequently awaken after a too-short nap may be overstimulated. Keep their waketime a little calmer.

Advantages to This Approach

By using this approach, you'll be able to schedule your day-to-day life more easily than if you follow on-demand or attachment parenting principles (see Chapter 12).

The "ignore it" approach doesn't assume that all parents are the same or parent in the same way. For example, some parents thrive on attachment parenting. Others do not. Considering the "ignore it" approach gives those parents another option. Parents who are more scheduled and dependent on routine will find that this approach suits their temperament better than parents who are more flexible and more child-centered.

Another advantage of the "ignore it" approach is that what's best for you—the needs of the parents—is as important as what's best for the baby. Since the demands of caring for a newborn can be overwhelming, having "permission" to think about yourself can help new parents get through the initial period of adjustment to their newborn. Recognizing that you need time alone, time with your spouse, and a good night's sleep—and providing for it—can help you deal with the demands of a baby.

 Melissa's Mindset

For a newborn, 2 hours between feedings (especially if the baby is being breastfed) is more typical than the 3 hours advocated in this approach. The American Academy of Pediatrics recommends that during the early weeks, breastfeeding infants be fed 8–12 times per 24 hours. Mothers are encouraged to feed the baby whenever she shows signs of hunger (rooting, mouthing, etc.).

Drawbacks to This Approach

The "ignore it" approach can seem rigid and cold to parents. The focus on schedules can seem inflexible. Many parents have difficulty ignoring the child's cries as he falls asleep, feeling like this is abandoning the baby or teaching the baby that parents can't be trusted to offer comfort. While some parents may find that the schedule gives them freedom, others feel that it makes them slaves to the clock. In addition, trying to wake the baby up after he has fallen asleep while feeding may be ineffective—he'll just fall asleep again. Finally, the 3-hour schedule may be too much time for an infant to go between feedings, especially a breast-fed child.

What Parents Say About This Approach

Many parents feel that some parts of this approach make a lot of sense—such as putting the baby down for the night at the same time every day—but that certain no-nos, such as never rocking your baby to sleep, are counterproductive or impossible to put into practice.

 Melissa's Mindset

Some babies are more amenable to this approach than others. In fact, some babies will never give a parent "trouble" with sleep from very early on, while others will have more difficulty putting themselves to sleep. Parents should remember to assess their own level of comfort with this approach as well as their knowledge of the child and what she needs when considering using this approach.

Some parents find that the approach works beautifully. Debbie used the "ignore it" method for her two children, now 2½ and 4½. "My older child was sleeping through the night by 10 weeks. At first she'd cry for 45 minutes at bedtime and then it gradually went down. She didn't respond to pats on the back or us coming back into the room, so we just let her wail. Stressful, to be sure, but nothing else worked for us." She waited until her second child was a little older—about 4 months old—before starting the "ignore it" method on him, and it worked just as well.

The Least You Need to Know

◆ Creating a stable schedule for your baby means less stress and fatigue for everyone.

◆ Using schedules to structure eating, waking, and sleeping allows the parent more control.

◆ Fitting your child into your schedule instead of allowing the child to dictate the schedule means each day is more predictable and routine.

◆ Ignoring your older baby's crying at sleeptime can help him learn to fall asleep by himself at bedtime and after night wakings.

Chapter 7

Pretend You Don't See Me

In This Chapter

- ◆ The "ignore but check" sleep-training approach
- ◆ How do you "Ferberize" your baby?
- ◆ Developing good sleep habits in your baby
- ◆ Creating comforting bedtime routines

An entire generation of parents has *Ferberized* their babies—that is, used the sleep-training methods of Dr. Richard Ferber to help teach their babies (and children) to fall asleep.

In this chapter, we'll discuss Dr. Ferber's method of gradually lengthening the amount of time you let your baby cry each night before checking on him. And we'll show you strategies you can use to help your baby fall asleep and stay asleep through the night.

We'll describe why bedtime routines are so important to babies and children and show you how you can develop a routine that suits your child. We'll also clue you in on what to avoid just before lights out (scary stories and tickling contests, anyone?).

"Ignore but Check" Approach

The "graduated extinction/systematic ignoring with minimal parental Check" approach (try saying that five times fast), as this approach is called by researchers, is a method of sleep training that uses some of the "ignore it" strategies (as described in Chapter 6), but is not as abrupt. In this method, you check in on your baby at gradually lengthening intervals.

To **Ferberize** is to use the graduated-extinction sleep-training methods of Dr. Richard Ferber to help your baby or child learn to sleep on his own.

In other words, you don't just ignore your baby until she finally falls asleep, exhausted and drained (not to mention the condition you'll be in). Instead, in gradually lengthening intervals, you check on the baby and reassure her that you're there. Maybe we could call it going "warm turkey" instead of "cold turkey."

Unhappy Baby Alert

With the forthcoming publication of the most recent revision of his work, Ferber has become a bit less dogmatic on this approach. He's now saying that his method is not the only method of sleep training, and for some children (anxious children, for example), this technique may actually be harmful. So even Dr. Ferber agrees that if this approach seems wrong for your baby, you should trust your instincts.

What It Is

In the "ignore but check" approach, you create a comforting bedtime routine for your baby or child and then leave her alone, while checking in occasionally—according to a progressive schedule—until the child falls asleep.

According to Ferber, even though most babies and children have brief wakings during the night, they can learn to fall back asleep on their own without any help from you.

- Begin by establishing a routine with your newborn, so that she can become accustomed to certain rituals at sleeptime.

- Consider having a more elaborate routine for nighttime so that your baby begins to understand that nighttime is different from naps that he takes during the day. For example, naptime could include a routine of a diaper change and a brief snuggle, whereas bedtime could include a warm bath, change into pajamas, a story, and then bed.

- Once your baby is about three months old, you can begin the process of letting him cry himself to sleep, checking on him at gradually longer intervals.

- Essentially, you'll put your baby down in his crib, tell him it's time to sleep, and leave the room. A few minutes later, if he is still crying, you check on him. Once you leave, you wait a slightly longer period of time before checking again.

Unhappy Baby Alert

Of course, a brand new baby who needs to be fed every few hours cannot and will not learn to fall back to sleep on his own without any help from you. You'll want to wait until your baby is a little older before using this method—at least 3 months old and possibly older than that.

Because babies can learn to *self-soothe* during those night wakings, you need to ignore the baby (or child) who cries and wants attention in the middle of the night using the same progressive checking approach as you use to help the baby fall asleep in the first place. This teaches the baby to learn to soothe himself back to sleep without you.

BABY BABBLE

Self-soothe is the ability for your baby to comfort himself so that he can fall asleep at bedtime and fall back to sleep after night wakings.

While you do let the baby or child "cry it out" when using this method, you check on him to reassure the child that you're there. You do this by checking at progressively longer intervals, both when the child is falling asleep at night and also when he awakens during the night.

Melissa's Mindset

According to Dr. Ferber, by 3 months, most babies can sleep through the night. Remember, however, that "sleeping through the night" won't happen for most babies throughout the first year of life. What Dr. Ferber means is that by 3 months of age, some babies can put themselves back to sleep after waking up so that *parents* can sleep through. Still, many researchers have found that typical babies don't regularly self-soothe until around 8 months of age.

And in This Corner: Supporters of This Approach

Infant Almanac

According to Dr. Ferber, most children have the ability to sleep well— that is, to fall asleep quickly at an appropriate time, to sleep through the night, and to wake at an appropriate time. So there is hope for you and your baby!

Dr. Richard Ferber is the best-known supporter of this approach, which he describes in his book, *Solve Your Child's Sleep Problems*. A sleep researcher and director of the Center for Pediatric Sleep Disorders at Children's Hospital, Boston, his theories are based on studies conducted in his sleep disorder clinic and in his clinical practice.

Using This Approach

Following the "ignore but check" approach requires you to …

♦ Insist that the child sleep alone.

♦ Develop a consistent, comforting bedtime routine.

♦ Offer and encourage attachment to a *transitional object*—a favorite toy, stuffed animal, or blanket.

BABY BABBLE

A **transitional object** is a favorite toy, stuffed animal, or blanket a young child can use to comfort herself while falling asleep (instead of relying on you to provide the comfort).

♦ Ignore crying for progressively longer periods of time before going to check on the child.

♦ Shut the door (and keep it shut) for progressively longer periods of time if your toddler refuses to stay in bed.

Sleeping Alone

Babies and children like to sleep with their parents, and many parents enjoy it, too. Among other things, it cuts down on bedtime arguments! But according to Ferber, studies have shown that such an arrangement disrupts your sleep as well as your child's.

Using this method doesn't mean that your child can never make the occasional visit to your bed. For instance, after a screaming nightmare or when the child has been sick, you may want to allow your child the additional comfort of sharing your bed. But routine co-sleeping may prevent parents from actually solving their child's sleep problems, according to Ferber.

For an alternative view about co-sleeping, see Chapter 12.

Infant Almanac

Ferber believes that sleeping alone helps the child learn to become an independent child (and eventually an independent adult), and contributes to his healthy psychological development.

Melissa's Mindset

Although many parents find solitary sleeping arrangements most beneficial, research shows that babies and children who sleep with their parent(s) do not suffer from psychological harm or dependency issues later in life.

Step-by-Step

For young infants, Ferber suggests feeding on demand and letting them develop their own sleep-wake routine based on their own schedule. This means feeding the baby when he appears hungry, and putting the baby to sleep when he appears drowsy.

Not all crying is hunger. You may be able to comfort your child and encourage sleep (without feeding her) by ...

- ◆ Walking the baby.
- ◆ Rocking the baby.
- ◆ Stroking the baby.

Unlike the strict "ignore it" supporters described in Chapter 6, Ferber believes that these comforting activities do not interfere with sleep training but actually reassure the newborn and help him fall asleep.

As your baby grows older, Ferber recommends increasing the amount of time between feedings so that eventually he is being fed every 3 hours or so (usually by age 3 months). Developing this schedule enables you to follow the baby's cues but lets you add structure to the routine.

By this age, Ferber says, most babies will be sleeping 5 to 9 hours at night. This is also the age where you can begin to use Ferber's "ignore but check" sleep-training method. (It will be ineffective on younger babies.)

Melissa's Mindset

Our research shows that most babies, on average, sleep about 5 hours at a time at night by 3 months. Some babies may sleep more or less than this amount, and this variability is normal.

Once the baby has developed this more consistent routine, parents should work to maintain it, according to Ferber. Thus, most days will take on a similar pattern. Again, you respond to your baby's cues but also develop a structure for her, instead of just reacting whenever the baby cries.

Parents of non-newborns begin this sleep-training method by developing a consistent, comforting bedtime routine.

A typical bedtime routine for a baby might include …

- Diaper change.
- Clothing change.
- Rocking while singing a lullaby.
- Putting the drowsy baby to bed in the crib.

For an older child (toddler age), the routine might include …

- Warm bath.
- Change into pajamas.
- Calm bedtime story.
- Brief tucking-in ritual.

What you *shouldn't* do is ...

- ◆ Read scary stories.

- ◆ Remind your child not to disturb the monsters under the bed.

- ◆ Play an energetic game of tag.

All of these activities will make it harder for your child to relax and fall asleep.

Ferber also recommends encouraging your child to attach to a transitional object like a toy or blanket. The object can be tucked into bed with the child and help comfort him as he falls asleep and when the child awakens throughout the night.

Checking On the Baby or Child

After your baby or child has been put to bed, Ferber's method requires that you let the child cry for a period of time before going in to check on her. So, for example, on the first day ...

Infant Almanac

According to Ferber, bedtime routines are important because sending the child off to bed alone can be scary for the child. By spending some personal time with the child before bed, she will be reassured and more likely to accept bedtime.

Melissa's Mindset

Research on infants' use of "transitional objects" or "sleep aids" finds that most babies use some type of object at the beginning of the night or in the middle of the night to help themselves fall asleep. It is not typically until after the first year, however, that a baby will attach to a specific object such as a "blankie" or a special stuffed animal.

- ◆ Wait five minutes before going in to check on the child.

- ◆ Extend the wait to 10 minutes before going to check on the child a second time.

- ◆ Wait 15 minutes before checking on the child for a third time.

- ◆ All subsequent checks require a waiting interval of 15 minutes.

On the second night, the intervals are a bit longer: 10 minutes for the first check, 15 for the second, 20 for the third and subsequent. By the seventh night, you wait 35 minutes before checking the child for the first time.

Use the same routine for when the child wakens during the night. Usually, it takes about a week for this approach to work, although it can take a little longer. If it does, simply add 5 more minutes to the waiting interval.

"Checking" the baby or child means going into the room to reassure the child, but spending only a few minutes with him. You don't rock, nurse, or hold the child (as you might a newborn), but rather, just pat him on the back or speak to him softly. You may need to lay the baby back down if he is standing in the crib.

Helping the Child Stay in Bed

While most of us can imagine making this method work when the baby is confined to a crib, what happens when the "baby" is a child who can climb out of bed? (And does!) You can't just ignore the crying then. You have to help your child learn to stay in bed, according to Ferber.

To do this, tell your child that she must stay in bed, and then close the bedroom door if the child does not stay in bed. Again, use a progressive method. For example, on the first night …

- ◆ Keep the door closed for 1 minute before going in and checking on the child.

- ◆ Wait 2 minutes before going in a second time.

- ◆ Extend the wait to 3 minutes before going in a third time.

- ◆ Wait 5 minutes before going in a fourth time and for each subsequent visit.

On the second day, lengthen the time by waiting 2 minutes for the first visit, 4 minutes for the second, and so on. By the seventh day, you're waiting 15 minutes before going in to check on the child. Again, this method usually takes about a week to work, but if it requires longer, just add a few minutes to the waiting interval.

Challenges You'll Encounter

Your ability to outlast your child is the main drawback to this method. Nerves of steel (not to mention a bottle of wine) help. A determined child can keep getting out of bed for hours, just as an overwrought baby can keep crying for hours. Giving in and rewarding the behavior now and then—*intermittent reinforcement*—helps you create a bigger problem.

Succumbing to the temptation of checking on the child earlier than indicated is the biggest challenge. It's important to be consistent when using the Ferber method. Going back and forth usually only results in your child crying even more. One slip and you've doubled the amount of time it will take for the baby to get back with the program.

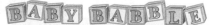

It definitely helps for you to have a partner to keep you honest, provide distraction, and hold your hand while waiting for the minutes to pass. Just be sure you're in agreement that you want to use the Ferber method before using it. Otherwise you'll be listening to your baby cry while also listening to your partner argue with you.

Intermittent reinforcement— responding *sometimes*—is the best way to *keep* a behavior happening.

Other challenges include the following:

◆ Children open doors. Just shutting the door won't keep most children in their room. You may have to play door cop, which can be unpleasant and make you feel uncomfortable. Holding the door shut while your toddler tries to open it usually does not improve your general disposition. Putting a gate up to prevent the child from leaving the room is an alternative, but care must be taken, as an agitated child could try to shove it out of the way or climb over it.

◆ Doing the technique at bedtime and during the middle of the night at the same time can be grueling. Plan on some major sleep deprivation for the first few nights at least (or consider trying the splitting it up" approach described in Chapter 9).

♦ After surviving the first night, you'll probably encounter even more unhappiness the next night. Resistance often gets worse before it gets better.

Advantages to This Approach

Creating a routine and sticking to it can help make living with your baby easier, more enjoyable, and less stressful. Other advantages include the following:

♦ Having the system in place helps you make decisions about your child. You don't have to wonder, "Should I go in and check on the baby?" All you have to do is look at the clock to know whether it's time.

♦ The "ignore but check" approach appeals to parents who want to establish a routine with their child but find the more abrupt "ignore it" approach (described in Chapter 6) too cold and lacking in compassion.

♦ If you can stick with it, the "graduated extinction" approach is highly effective in teaching a child to sleep on his own.

Drawbacks to This Approach

The "ignore but check" approach is supposed to keep the baby's crying to a minimum, but in some cases it actually makes the baby cry more. This is because you do soothe the baby periodically, so she may develop the habit of just crying until you show up (which you eventually will).

Sensitive parents may find this approach aversive; listening to a baby cry is difficult and may be too much for many parents to take.

What Parents Say About This Approach

Jen took up the "ignore but check" approach out of desperation. "My younger son was 'The Thing That Wouldn't Sleep.' He got into bad sleep habits from the start, first with colic and then with reflux, both of which made him miserable," she says. "So, he got used to being soothed, and didn't learn to soothe himself back to sleep."

As many parents find, Jen learned that getting her baby to sleep usually wasn't the problem—the problem was *keeping* him asleep.

"He'd wake up several times a night until he was 16 months old. I'd had enough!" So she tried Ferber's "ignore but check" approach. "It worked! He slept through the night rather well after that, except for a few setbacks whenever he got a cold.

"Here's my tip: Start it and stick to it as early as possible. The younger they are, the easier it is." Because her son was old enough to get out of bed, the whole process was that much more difficult. He had to be kept in his room at the same time Jen was trying to teach him to soothe himself to sleep. This approach is definitely easier with a younger baby (although many parents wait until they are desperate to try it).

The Least You Need to Know

- ◆ "Ignore but check" is slightly less severe than the "ignore it" approach.

- ◆ Using progressively longer periods between checks on your child encourages him to fall asleep on his own.

- ◆ Using the bedroom door as a means to control access (instead of yelling at the child or continually scooping her up and putting her back in bed) means you can help the child learn to stay in bed.

- ◆ This method can work with any age child.

Chapter 8

Being Seen but Not Heard

In This Chapter

- The "ignore it but be there" sleep-training approach
- Helping your baby learn to self-soothe
- Changing negative sleep associations to positive ones
- Learning to ignore unwanted sleep behaviors to help eliminate them

"Not a creature was stirring ... not even a mouse." That's every parent's fond dream—but the reality is that babies and young children do a lot of stirring while they're trying to get to sleep and stay asleep.

In this chapter we'll show how the "ignore it but be there" approach to sleep training can help you settle your little mouse down for a long winter's night.

"Ignore It But Be There" Approach

According to Jodi A. Mindell, one of the best-known supporters of this method, 25 percent of young children experience sleep problems, including sleep disruptions, difficulty falling asleep, and difficulty staying asleep. So plenty of desperate parents out there are looking for answers to sleep problems.

One of the basic building blocks of the "ignore it but be there" approach is that ignoring bad behavior causes it to go away. (Now if only the same thing could be said of credit card bills!) If you don't "reinforce" undesirable behavior by responding to it (even negative attention is a reinforcer), then the child will eventually find some other, one hopes more positive, way of getting attention.

> **Infant Almanac**
>
> Breast-fed babies typically sleep for shorter periods of time and are usually older when they begin to sleep through the night than formula-fed babies.

In this method, you begin encouraging good sleep habits by developing a bedtime routine as soon as you bring your baby home from the hospital. Once your baby is about six weeks old, you establish a schedule for him. Later, when your baby is four to six months old, you can start allowing him to cry it out for short periods of time.

What It Is

The approach has three main steps:

- ◆ Develop a sleep schedule.
- ◆ Create a bedtime routine.
- ◆ Put the baby down while drowsy but awake.
- ◆ Stay close by—even in the same room—but let the baby cry to settle himself to sleep.

It is important to separate feeding from sleep, and you want to teach your baby to soothe herself back to sleep.

And in This Corner: Supporters of This Approach

One of the main supporters of this approach, Jodi A. Mindell, Ph.D., is associate director of the Sleep Center at the Children's Hospital of Philadelphia. Her classic book, *Sleeping Through the Night*, is based on her research and on parental anecdotes.

Using This Approach

Age 6 weeks is an ideal time to begin to establish a good sleep schedule. Establishing the schedule early prevents later sleep difficulties. Physically, most babies are able to sleep for longer continuous periods of time once they've reached this age.

Using this approach, you'll set a regular schedule and routine for bedtimes. You'll help your child learn to soothe herself back to sleep (offering comfort when she's unable to do so) and be firm in not rewarding unwanted behavior. For example, you may pat your child on her back to encourage her to settle down (offering comfort), but you won't take her out of the bed and let her stay up later just because she's fussing (rewarding unwanted behavior).

Infant Almanac

You can lead a baby to bed but you can't make her sleep. That's okay. Just put her to bed when it's bedtime. For young babies up to a year or so, you may have to rock and soothe, but for older children, such as toddlers, you'll want to be firm in setting limits. They don't have to sleep but they have to remain quietly in their bed when it's naptime or bedtime.

Step-by-Step

Start by creating a routine for naptime and bedtime. For bedtime, this might be a bath, a change of diaper and clothes, and a song; for naptime it might be a shorter routine, such as a change of diaper and a song. This can be done with a newborn.

Next, establish a sleep schedule. This includes …

◆ The same bedtime every night.

Infant Almanac

All babies wake during the night, but many can be trained to soothe themselves back to sleep without your intervention. Many parents are surprised at how their children can soothe themselves if they're allowed to try. Babies who can't soothe themselves may need to be rocked or nursed back to sleep.

Infant Almanac

Usually when you use this method, you sit in the room until your baby falls asleep, but another approach calls for the parent to sleep in the same room as the baby for 1 week while completely ignoring the fussing. Your presence is supposed to calm the baby even though you don't make eye or verbal contact with her or take her out of the crib.

◆ The same waketime every morning.

◆ Set naptimes.

Naptimes are based on a set feeding schedule of about every 2 hours. This step will work best if your baby is at least 6 weeks old.

Most important is teaching your child to soothe himself. This is why putting the baby down while he is drowsy but still awake is important. You can put your baby down drowsy but still awake at any time, but ignoring the unwanted behavior (i.e., the crying) should wait until the child is older (at least four months).

Realize that with a young baby (6 weeks or so) you're just "practicing" this approach. At 6 weeks, your baby is too young to be allowed to cry for long periods of time. Here's what to do:

◆ Try the steps as described. Your baby may fall asleep without too much fussing. Hooray!

◆ If not, don't fret. Just do what you normally do to help your child fall asleep.

◆ Try again during the next sleep period.

Creating Positive Sleep Associations

A fundamental principle in the "ignore it but be there" approach is to help your baby develop appropriate sleep associations so he can learn to fall asleep on his own. Actually, establishing positive sleep associations is important for almost every approach discussed in this book.

We all have certain rituals we do before falling asleep. We associate certain things with bedtime—and with sleep. Maybe we have milk and cookies, take a warm bath, turn around in a circle three times (no, wait, that's the dog). If we aren't able to do our rituals—we're on vacation, in the hospital, or on the sofa after losing an argument—we have trouble sleeping.

Unhappy Baby Alert

Many babies wake and want a feeding just as Mom and Dad are drifting off to dreamland. This can cause tears all around. Instead, try waking your baby before you go to sleep and giving her a "parents' bedtime" feeding. The baby will probably be happy to eat and will fall back asleep, ready to let you hit the pillow for 3 or 4 hours. Ah, bliss!

The same thing is true of babies and children. So you want to encourage positive sleep associations. For one child this might be a favorite blanket, a night-light on, and the door closed. If you ensure that those associations are there all the time, your baby will have an easier time of falling asleep—and of falling back asleep after she wakes up.

Melissa's Mindset

Remember that the key is to make everything that happens when the baby falls asleep the same when the baby wakes up in the middle of the night. So, if you play music for baby at bedtime, that music should be playing throughout the night. The trick is to make the environment as constant as possible. Pacifiers are helpful for some babies, but before they are able to find and replace that binky on their own in the middle of the night, prepare to be the designated "binky-replacer."

Negative sleep associations are things that won't be there should your baby wake up in the middle of the night. That includes you. So if your baby relies on you to fall asleep, then of course she's going to demand you when she wakes up in the middle of the night. If you can create positive sleep associations (i.e., things that are not you and don't require your presence), then your baby or child is more likely to fall back to sleep without needing your presence.

Sleep Issues as Your Baby Grows

As your baby grows, his sleep associations will also change. In some cases, you'll have to help him develop new sleep associations in order to reduce the amount of disrupted sleep he gets (not to mention you!).

> **Infant Almanac**
>
> Research shows that negative sleep associations are a primary reason for sleep problems in young children. So making the associations positive can eliminate or prevent many sleep problems in children.

For example, babies outgrow the need for feedings in the middle of the night but may still wake at feeding time. You may need to substitute something else for the feeding. A partner can be helpful in breaking the "feed-sleep" association by taking over nighttime soothing. Then, when it is time to have a bottle or breastfeed in the morning, the parent should tell the baby, "It's time." Drawing the curtains or turning on a light could be a signal. The baby will learn to associate this signal with feeding. When the signal isn't there in the middle of the night, she'll know not to expect a feeding.

As your baby becomes a toddler, you may also notice an increase in night wakings. Again, this is because of cognitive and motor growth in your toddler. Your toddler may not be able to soothe himself back to sleep and may require some soothing from you. Again, you may need to change associations so your child can soothe himself back to sleep.

Also around this age, children start to resist going to bed. They're becoming more independent and want more control over themselves. (This is no news to parents of a toddler!) They may also think you save all the fun stuff until after they go to bed. Little do they know you're paying the bills and clipping your toenails. Again, discourage the unwanted behavior and encourage positive sleep associations. Re-establish your "ignore it but be there" approach if needed.

Children around this age may also start having nightmares and fears. These are normal. Your child may need reassurance, but you will also need to set limits on how much attention can be demanded. (See Chapter 16 for more information on coping with toddler sleep difficulties.)

Dealing with Sleep Issues

Even though you may notice more sleep problems as your child gets older, you will continue to use many of the same strategies as you did when the child was a newborn. Here are some examples:

◆ Maintain regular naptimes and bedtimes.

◆ Create a bedtime routine appropriate to an older child.

◆ Continue to put your child to sleep drowsy but awake.

In addition, the following strategies are important for dealing with older children, such as toddlers:

◆ Create a consistent bedroom environment—objects should be in the same place all the time.

◆ Maintain a cool, quiet, dark, and comfortable bedroom environment.

◆ Set consistent, reasonable limits and enforce them.

◆ Try a transitional object (security device) like a stuffed toy or a blanket.

And don't forget to warn your child about transitions: "It's 10 minutes until bedtime," for example. This helps the child make the mental adjustment from play to bedtime routine.

When sleep problems have reared their ugly head, sometimes parents need to use some form of "ignoring" as discussed in Chapters 6 and 7. Consider using the "ignore but be there" method. What's different about this technique is that parents stay in the room while asking the baby to stay in his crib.

> **Infant Almanac**
>
> Use a timer to help your child transition from play to bedtime routine. Let your child know that she has 10 minutes before bedtime. When the timer goes off, it's time for the bedtime routine.

For example, parents may sit in a chair next to the crib until baby falls asleep on night one, then move the chair a few inches toward the door on night two, and then move the chair farther on night three, and so on. Eventually, the parent is out of the room, and the negative sleep association has been broken without too many tears on anyone's part.

Challenges You'll Encounter

Creating and maintaining a set schedule is sometimes challenging. Also, there's a fine line between helping soothe your child to sleep and making your child dependent on you. Using this method, that line is not clearly drawn—it depends on you and your baby. So you can sometimes actually create sleep problems without realizing it. As long as you remember to always end the routine with baby or child drowsy but not fully asleep when put to bed, these problems can be avoided.

Melissa's Mindset

A "cool, quiet, dark, and comfortable bedroom environment" means that parents should rethink the TV and VCR that are installed in junior's bedroom. Children who have TVs in their rooms have been found to get less sleep. Keep the TV in the family room and avoid this sleep-gobbler. Remember, more sleep equals a happier, healthier child (and parents)!

Also, as your child grows older, setting and enforcing firm limits can be difficult. Not responding to unwanted behavior takes a lot of patience—and self-confidence!

Once the child moves from the crib into a bed, this technique becomes more work. Parents would be best advised to start establishing healthy sleep habits early, before the little cherub becomes an accomplished bed escapee.

Parents with hectic, erratic schedules may find it difficult to establish the consistent routines needed for this approach.

Advantages to This Approach

This method appeals to many parents who feel that schedules are important but who do not want to leave their babies to cry it out. It enable s them the flexibility to respond to their baby's needs on any particular day instead of letting the schedule take precedence.

The approach can be used through-out a child's life, and the method of ignoring unwanted bedtime behav-ior can be used to deal with any unwanted behavior, during the day or night.

Melissa's Mindset

In one of the rare research studies into sleep-training techniques, Karen France found that this approach worked best in getting babies to sleep and reducing crying, compared to complete ignoring and ignoring but checking.

Drawbacks to This Approach

Does going in to soothe the baby tonight count as appropriate parental presence, or does it just encourage unwanted behavior? Without clear lines of distinction, parents can feel that they're not sure if their behav-ior is helping or hindering the child's sleep habits.

What Parents Say About This Approach

Jennifer successfully used this approach (and continues to use it) with her daughter. Although not a schedule-lover herself, she quickly real-ized that her baby did much better going to sleep at the same time every night, getting up at the same time every morning, and having naps and feeding times at about the same time every day.

"When the baby had an off day or seemed hungrier or more tired than usual, I'd accommodate," says Jennifer. "So it wasn't 'live or die by the schedule.' I might have a plan for the day, but I'd adjust if it looked like she wasn't going to get enough sleep during naptime and was therefore going to be a cranky terror at the grocery store."

Her daughter was very quick to pick up on self-soothing methods, and by her toddler years would put herself to sleep with little help from her parents. On those few occasions when she seemed fussy or battled her parents about bedtime, her parents just ignored the behavior, put her back in bed if she'd gotten out, and didn't make a fuss. Soon she real-ized that she wasn't getting anything from her efforts and went back to being an easy kid to put to bed.

As she grew older, she had occasional sleep problems during transitions, such as her parents' divorce, starting school, and after hospitalizations.

"When that happened, I thought it was fine for me to help soothe her back to sleep, even when she was an older preschooler," says Jennifer. "I sang lots of lullabies, gave lots of back massages. Once in a while she'd wind up in bed with me if that seemed to be the best way to help her feel secure. But we stuck to the schedule as best we could and when I felt that she was ready, I would tell her that she needed to go to bed and that I would ignore her fussing if she didn't go to bed. That always worked."

It even worked when Jessica began having sleep problems at age 8. "At first I was so surprised at her having sleep problems that I handled it poorly—threats and punishment," says Jennifer. "Then I realized that I needed to do what had always worked—stick to a routine schedule throughout the day and evening, maintain a set bedtime and wake-time, encourage a bedtime routine—and at her age, it was all stuff that she could manage on her own except the final goodnight kiss. Then I vowed to ignore the behavior instead of responding to it in any way. We had a sharp increase in her challenges at bedtime right at first but I ignored them and she stopped within 2 weeks."

Jennifer swears by the system and plans to continue to use it should future sleep problems crop up.

The Least You Need to Know

♦ Babies need routine—set sleep and waketimes, and set bedtime routines.

♦ Teaching your baby to soothe himself to sleep is the most important strategy in your sleep-training arsenal.

♦ Every baby is different, so your approach needs to be responsive to your baby's needs.

♦ Ignoring your baby's fussing and crying but being there for him can help him learn to soothe himself to sleep.

♦ Ignoring unwanted behavior eliminates the behavior.

Chapter 9

Splitting It Up

In This Chapter

- The "splitting it up" sleep-training approach
- Setting the stage for bedtime
- Dealing with night wakings only after the baby is able to fall asleep on his own
- How to "Ferberize" your baby in a kinder, gentler way

Your baby may weigh less than 20 pounds, but she can put up a fight that could make a grown adult cry. That's especially true when it comes to sleep. It may *seem* simple to us—go to bed, fall asleep, get up in the morning, and go to work. But it's not so simple for your baby, and that means it's not so simple for you. Your baby has to learn how to fall asleep and stay asleep, just as you once did.

By now you know that getting your baby to fall asleep at bedtime is only half the battle. Getting your baby to sleep through the night—or at least to fall back asleep without your help after he wakes at night—is the other half. In this chapter, we'll describe one approach that says, "Fight half the battle first, and the other half will follow."

In this chapter, we'll explain how tackling one problem at a time can eliminate both problems while enabling you to retain your sanity and maybe even get a little sleep.

Ignoring at Bedtime; Ignoring in the Middle of the Night

Using this approach, you deal with bedtime sleep problems first. Once bedtime is established and the baby is putting herself to sleep without much fuss, then you deal with the middle of the night awakenings.

The "splitting it up" approach uses steps similar to the "ignore but check" method, described in Chapter 7—letting the child fuss for progressively longer periods of time—but you don't deal with bedtime and night wakings at the same time. This means you're stricter in how you handle bedtime, and more flexible about how you respond to nighttime wakings (again, at first). Later, you will deal with night wakings more systematically if you need to. (And you may not need to.)

What It Is

The "splitting it up" approach is two-fold and fairly straightforward. In phase 1, you …

- Establish bedtime first and get baby to fall asleep on his own on a regular basis, using ignore methods (see Chapters 7 and 8).
- Do whatever works for nighttime wakings.

Simple as that.

Of course, nothing involving babies is ever as simple as that. But sometimes, babies who are trained using this method do get the hint after you've done these first two steps. As a result, say supporters of the method, they have fewer nighttime wakings.

The idea is that your baby will learn to fall asleep by herself at bedtime, and that such training will eventually help her fall asleep again when she wakes at night. In other words, she will learn the self-soothing behaviors she needs to put herself back to sleep after night wakings.

Thus she will naturally need your help less and less as you continue to teach her how to fall asleep at bedtime. But instead of having to listen to her cry it out when she wakes at night, you can comfort her in whatever way makes sense to you.

If, after a few weeks, the baby continues to have nighttime wakings despite using this method, you move into phase 2. Phase 2 involves following the same ignore method that you used to teach the baby to fall asleep on her own at the beginning of the night—only now you use the method for the middle-of-the-night wakings.

> **Infant Almanac**
>
> Phase 2 of this method is done only after your baby can successfully put himself to sleep at the beginning of the night without too much fuss.

Melissa's Mindset

Research conducted by Berndt Eckerberg, a sleep researcher, shows that babies whose parents help them learn to fall asleep on their own at the beginning of the night often teach themselves to fall back to sleep upon awakening in the middle of the night without any need for phase 2. However, many parents report that their babies continue to wake up at night after successfully putting themselves to sleep at bedtime. Parents choosing this method should be prepared to move into phase 2 after giving the child a couple of weeks to get the hang of self-soothing.

And in This Corner: Supporters of This Approach

One of the main supporters of this approach, Dr. Berndt Eckerberg, is a researcher in Sweden whose clinical study of this two-part sleep-training method showed that most of the babies who were trained this way woke up less frequently and cried less often (as compared to other ignore methods).

Jodi Mindell, Ph.D, a supporter of the "ignore but be there" approach described in Chapter 8, also thinks that this approach can work for parents, believing that if you deal with bedtime, sometimes nighttime will follow without any extra assistance.

Using This Approach

First things first. You can start by establishing a bedtime routine so that the baby knows it's nighttime and time to sleep as soon as your baby's born. But you won't be able to establish a regular bedtime or start the ignoring/checking part of the process until your baby is around 3 months old. A bedtime routine should include a regular bedtime and a calm, dark, and quiet sleep environment, and may include a bath, a feeding, diaper change, clothing change, and a lullaby (maybe a story if the baby is older).

Melissa's Mindset

For parents who are interested in doing the "ignore but check" method (see Chapter 7), the "splitting it up" approach is a more pleasant way to go, since you aren't committed to changing everything at once. But you also run the risk of confusing the baby, who might start waking up more after being put to bed to get that nighttime attention from her parents.

Once you have a routine in place, you use the "ignore but check" method described in Chapter 7 to train your baby to fall asleep on her own. If you prefer a gentler approach, you can instead use one of the modified extinction methods, such as the "ignore it but be there" approach to deal with bedtime (see Chapter 8 for more information about this method).

Step-by-Step

For phase 1 of this program, you focus only on getting your baby to fall asleep on her own at bedtime. To do this …

- ◆ Create a soothing bedtime routine (as described above).

- ◆ Put your baby to bed awake (drowsy helps).

- ◆ If your child fusses, give brief *verbal contact* every 5 minutes until he stops fussing and goes to sleep.

- ◆ On following nights, stay away for progressively longer intervals.

- ◆ Do whatever you want to comfort baby during night wakings.

Within a week, your baby should be fussing less and be able to put herself to sleep at bedtime. If it takes a few days longer, that's fine. Just continue to lengthen the checking-up-on-her interval. If your baby is still having trouble falling asleep after several weeks of training, you will want to double-check that you're following the procedure correctly.

Once you've established bedtime and your baby is falling asleep without your help, you may find that he is able to put himself back to sleep if he wakes during the night. If this doesn't happen naturally, you move into phase 2 of "splitting it up."

> **BABY BABBLE**
>
> A **verbal contact** means using words to soothe the baby rather than picking him up, nursing him, and so on. "Mama's here," "Hush, baby, time for sleep," and the like, let the baby know you're there but encourage him to fall asleep without more active intervention.

Phase 2

For phase 2, you use the same approach to deal with night wakings as you did to settle your baby down for bedtime in phase 1:

- Check on baby.

- Give verbal reassurance.

- Leave.

- If baby still fusses, return in 5 minutes.

- Allow progressively longer periods between checks.

Again, this may take a week or so to work. Just continue to lengthen the interval between checks. While the "splitting it up" method takes longer than the "ignore but check" method used alone, if you're not making progress after several weeks, you may want to reassess. Your baby may be too young to benefit from the training. Trying again after a month or so has elapsed may help, or you may want to review what you're doing to ensure that you're following the training method appropriately.

> **Infant Almanac**
>
> Some babies will get the point once you train them how to fall asleep on their own at bedtime and won't need further help to fall asleep after night wakings.

Using the Method with Older Babies

If your child is old enough to get out of the crib or out of bed, the approach is modified slightly.

During phase 1:

◆ The parent sits outside the baby's room, not paying any attention to the child.

◆ If the child leaves his bed, the parent puts the child back to bed without comment.

◆ This continues until the child falls asleep.

See Chapter 8 for other tips on dealing with sleep training older babies who can get out of bed on their own.

Once the child is able to fall asleep at bedtime without parental help, he may be able to soothe himself to sleep after night wakings without your help. If he still has night wakings after learning to put himself to sleep at bedtime, you can use this same method at night. During phase 2, if your older baby gets out of bed during a night waking, simply put him back to bed without comment.

Infant Almanac

Because of the additional challenges of sleep training an older infant who can (and will!) climb out of bed, you may want to consider sleep training your baby when she is a bit younger and less mobile. Even so, Eckerberg believes that you should only begin sleep training if you feel that your baby has a sleep problem (or if you have a sleep problem because of your baby's sleep habits)—which may not be apparent until the baby is older.

Challenges You'll Encounter

Just as with the "ignore but check" method described in Chapter 7, your ability to put up with fussing from your child is the main difficulty here. A determined baby can cry for a long time!

Just as with other ignore methods, some parents find it too difficult to let their babies cry it out.

Another challenge with this method is that the baby may fall asleep fine at bedtime but then wake up more at night to get the anything-goes contact from parents.

Melissa's Mindset

I've seen babies fall asleep perfectly fine on their own, then need a parent after an hour of sleep, and then throughout the night. My sister experienced this and needed to teach her son to soothe himself for nighttime wakings using "ignore but check," even though he was perfectly capable of falling asleep on his own at bedtime.

Advantages to This Approach

Again, just as with the "ignore but check" method described in Chapter 7, having a clear system in place reduces doubt and questions about what you should be doing.

With this approach, you're only dealing with one issue of sleep training at a time—bedtime first, and then night wakings. This can make the battle seem easier to fight. And it might be less stressful for parents to know that they don't need to tackle the whole night at once.

Parents can continue to soothe their baby however they wish during the middle of the night when the baby wakes up, so they may get more sleep … at least at first.

Drawbacks to This Approach

Dealing with sleep problems at bedtime only may encourage the baby to wake more at night, which is not the goal of most parents!

Also, it may be difficult as a parent (not to mention how it might be confusing for your baby) to follow two different approaches at night: ignore at bedtime but then comfort however you want at night wakings. You may start to question why you can't just do what works at bedtime, too.

For parents who find the "ignore but check" approach difficult to begin with, this approach may make things worse by prolonging the pain. At least with traditional ignoring but checking you are promised a sleeping baby within a week or so. Splitting it up will definitely take longer if your baby is still waking up at night after self-soothing at bedtime.

What Parents Say About This Approach

Julie knew she wanted to try the "ignore but check" method even before her first child was born (after hearing parent horror stories of babies never falling asleep). She and her husband read Ferber's classic book, *Solve Your Child's Sleep Problems*, and for them, "The big take-away that we followed was: Let your baby learn to put herself to sleep. [Ferber] totally convinced us that 'rocking a baby to sleep' or otherwise trying to 'help' was setting yourself up for big problems."

So with both of their children, Julie and her husband would put them down in their own beds, awake, according to a routine. "Consequently, we did not fight a lot of battles at bedtime," she says.

However, she found trying to use Ferber's "ignore but check" method for night wakings too difficult, especially when the babies were young. That was when she decided to do what worked during the middle of the night ("It was purely sleep deprivation driving it," she says). Often she and the baby would just end up falling asleep in bed together. "As they were able to sleep through the night, it ceased to be an issue," she explains. She never had to go back to using Ferber in the middle of the night.

She recommends the approach to all parents. "We have friends who got wrapped up in helping their kids fall asleep [and they] have continued to struggle with sleep issues," she says. "We never really did, and I'm convinced it was largely because of this policy."

The Least You Need to Know

- ◆ "Splitting it up" enables you to work on getting the baby to fall asleep at bedtime before also tackling night wakings.

- ◆ Once you train your child to fall asleep on his own at bedtime, he may not need any further training to fall asleep after night wakings.

- ◆ Using progressively longer periods between checks on your child encourages her to fall asleep on her own.

- ◆ "Splitting it up" is a gentler way to use the "ignore but check" method with your child.

Part

3

No More Tears

If you can't stand the thought of letting your baby cry herself to sleep, then you'll want to consider a sleep-training approach that reduces the need for tears.

In this part, we'll show you a variety of tried-and-true methods for helping your child learn to sleep without tears—and without becoming completely sleep deprived yourself.

Chapter

10

Wake My Baby Up?
Are You Insane?

In This Chapter

- The "scheduled awakenings" sleep-training approach

- How waking your baby up before he wakes himself up can help him learn to sleep through the night

- Using progressively longer periods of time between wakings to encourage longer periods of sleep

- Waking your child up can eliminate the need to listen to a crying child

It's the middle of the night. The baby is sleeping soundly in her crib. You walk into her room, smile down at her sweet face—and wake her up.

No, we're not crazy. In this chapter, we'll explain how to use the "scheduled awakenings" approach to sleep training in order to help your child learn to sleep through the night. We'll show how keeping track of her usual wakings will help you identify her waking pattern, and how putting yourself in control of her wakings can help her learn to sleep through the night.

The "Scheduled Awakenings" Approach

This method is used for babies and children who don't have a problem settling at bedtime, but who do wake frequently through the night. Using this method, you put the baby to bed at bedtime, using whatever approach you have chosen to encourage him to fall asleep by himself. Or you may be one of the lucky ones with a baby who falls asleep at the beginning of the night without any fuss and without any encouragement from you. Hey, it could happen.

To deal with night wakings, you wake the baby before he wakes up himself, gradually increasing the length of time between awakenings until the baby is sleeping through the night. You don't need to keep the baby awake long—just long enough to be sure he's awake. Then let him go back to sleep, which he most likely will because he's drowsy. If not, soothe him in whatever way works. You can feed him or do whatever comforts him to help him get back to sleep. The waking-up process interrupts his night waking pattern and may help him learn how to soothe himself back to sleep.

Melissa's Mindset

The "scheduled awakenings" method has been shown in some research to be as effective as the extinction methods (see Chapters 6, 7, and 8) but doesn't involve the withdrawal of parents' attention at night. This means it doesn't cause the baby to cry during nighttime wakings, a big plus for many parents.

Remember, this approach is only used to treat night-waking issues, not settling. So if the baby settles fine but wakes up frequently, you may want to consider using the "scheduled awakenings" approach. But if you can't get the baby settled down at bedtime, then you will need to try another approach first to solve that problem.

What It Is

Many babies and children who wake at night do so at consistent times from one night to the next. The "scheduled awakenings" approach calls for you to keep track of your child's nighttime wakings for a period of time (usually several days to a week).

Once you know your child's typical waking pattern, you wake her up about 15 to 30 minutes before her usual wake time. Then you soothe

the baby back to sleep using whatever method you feel most comfortable with. Because you woke her up, she's tired and should fall back to sleep without too much trouble. The important part is that the parent starts getting control over the wakings so they don't happen spontaneously.

The basic idea is that the child will not then wake at her usual time (so we hope, anyway). Soon the night wakings are under the parent's control—they do the waking up; the baby doesn't wake up by herself. Eventually, the parent lengthens the amount of time between wakings until the baby is sleeping for longer and longer periods of time—and eventually sleeping through the entire night. Because waking up in the middle of the night is considered necessary and normal for very young infants, experts recommend starting the "scheduled awakenings" approach no earlier than 3–4 months.

And in This Corner: Supporters of This Approach

Avi Sadeh, a sleep researcher, discusses this method in his book, *Sleeping Like a Baby*. Many other sleep researchers, such as Brett Kuhn, agree that it can be an effective method for reducing night wakings.

Using This Approach

The "scheduled awakenings" approach requires a commitment by the parents to follow the process faithfully for up to 2 months (it can take that long to get rid of the nighttime wakings completely). In other words, you'll need to invest in an industrial-strength alarm clock to wake you up throughout the night so that you can, in turn, wake up the baby!

Scheduled awakenings will not involve too many extra awakenings on your part, because you are waking the baby just before he would naturally awaken anyway. You soothe the baby as you normally would. If you have a child with night-waking issues, you know the drill! The only difference is that *you* are waking the child instead of vice versa.

 Melissa's Mindset

This approach is for parents who have babies or young children who wake up during the night and who want to help their babies sleep through the night without having to withdraw attention (as is required by any of the "extinction" methods).

Step-by-Step

Begin by keeping a sleep log, such as the one on the following page, noting the times during the night that your baby wakes up. After about a week, you'll see the trend: your baby probably wakes up at consistent times from night to night. Those are her established night-waking times.

Next, when you're ready to begin the program, you put your baby to sleep at bedtime using whatever method you're accustomed to. Then set your alarm for about 15 to 30 minutes before your baby's first typical night waking. While your baby is still asleep, gently wake him up. Once he is roused, soothe him back to sleep using whatever method works. There is no need to keep the baby awake—you just need to see the whites of his eyes and then help him to get back to sleep (if necessary). Yes, yes, we know it sounds insane. But it's effective in many cases. In fact, research has shown that this technique is as effective as the "ignore it" techniques discussed in Chapters 6 and 7.

Melissa's Mindset

Remember that this approach is not designed to help babies and children with bedtime-settling difficulties. If you are using this approach, your baby goes to bed without a problem; it's the night waking that's driving you insane. That's why there are no regulations about bedtime with this approach. It assumes that your child has no problems going to bed.

After you wake the baby, he will typically fall asleep quickly because he's still tired. And in most cases he won't wake at his usual scheduled time because you have already woken him up. Think of it like this: your child has established some regular times of night waking (say, at midnight, 3:30 A.M., and 5 A.M.). You wake the child up at 11:45 P.M., 3:15 A.M., and 4:45 A.M. Thus, there is no need for the child to wake up on his own. You've already taken care of the comforting that he has grown accustomed to at these times.

Night-Waking Sleep Log

	Day 1	Day 2	Day 3	Day 4	Day 5	Day 6	Day 7
Time to bed							
Time baby fell asleep							
Time of first night waking							
Back to sleep							
Time of second night waking							
Back to sleep							
Time of third night waking							
Back to sleep							
Time of fourth night waking							
Back to sleep							
Morning wake-time							

Continue waking the baby about 15 minutes to half an hour before his typical night wakings for the rest of the night—and for the next several nights.

The baby will most likely still have some *spontaneous awakenings* at first. Even though you took good notes and thought you had the pattern down, the baby may throw a curve ball and wake up at 2:00 A.M. in addition to his regular midnight, 3:30 A.M., and 5:00 A.M. pattern.

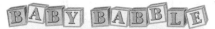

> **Spontaneous awakenings** are times when the baby wakes on his own, without your help. The goal of the "scheduled awakenings" approach is to get rid of the spontaneous awakenings.

No need to despair. Soothe the baby and continue waking him before the remainder of his typical waking times. After about a week, the baby will stop waking up at these extra times, say supporters of this approach. Congratulations! You are now in control of the baby's waking times.

> **Infant Almanac**
>
> If the baby wakes up spontaneously, soothe her back to sleep as you typically would, and continue waking her up before each of her subsequent typical awakening times.

Once the baby's spontaneous awakenings have gone away, start gradually increasing the time between wakings. So in the second week, for example, you might wake the baby up twice per night instead of three times. In subsequent weeks, you wake the baby only once and eventually you don't wake her at all. By taking control of the waking times, you have taught the baby to sleep through the night. This process can take from 4 to 8 weeks, depending on the baby.

Troubleshooting

If your baby doesn't have any discernable wake pattern, you will find the "scheduled awakenings" approach more difficult to use. That doesn't mean it can't be done! It will just be more challenging. Consider the following before implementing the "scheduled awakenings" program if your child has erratic awakenings:

◆ Your baby may be too young to benefit from sleep training. Waiting a few weeks may make all the difference.

◆ Take a break and then try keeping the log for a different week. It could be that your baby was just experiencing overtiredness, disruption from a vacation or a visit with relatives, or the like.

◆ Try putting the baby down at the same time every night. This might help you see the pattern.

If none of these ideas makes a difference, try "averaging" the waketimes that you've recorded in the sleep log. For example, while your child may not wake up precisely at midnight every night, you may spot a cluster of waketimes around that period—for example, on Monday your baby woke at 11:30, on Tuesday at 12:15, on Wednesday at 11:00, on Thursday at midnight, and so on. In that case, it would make sense to schedule one of your wakings for midnight.

> **Infant Almanac**
>
> If your child has no clear pattern, you may deal with more spontaneous awakenings than you would with a child who has more regular waketimes, but with patience you will be able to make this method work.

Challenges You'll Encounter

Some parents just cannot get used to the idea of waking a sleeping baby. If this is you, you may find it easier to commit to the program if you discuss it with your baby's pediatrician and get the reassurance you need that the program will probably work for you and your child.

Another challenge is that the method can take a while to work. Which means …

◆ You may be interrupted in the process with illness, vacation, visits from grandma, and the like.

◆ You may stop being consistent—it is difficult to get up to wake your baby, night after night.

◆ You may give up and go to bed.

Also, parents will need to set an alarm for themselves to wake up so that they can wake up the baby, sometimes several times per night, depending on how severe the night waking is. This might wake up an otherwise sleeping partner and end up causing more household sleep disruption at first. Other family members may be able to sleep through the baby's cries, but it's harder to ignore an alarm clock!

Some babies do not wake up at the same time every night, so it can be difficult to find a pattern to follow. It will take even longer for parents to use this approach with such a baby.

Advantages to This Approach

The "scheduled awakenings" approach works as well as the extinction methods do to get rid of night wakings, but you don't have to listen to your baby crying or withdraw your attention during the night. So in that sense it's easier on your nerves.

This approach is helpful to committed parents who want to take control of their children's awakenings and teach them to sleep through the night while still being able to soothe them as they want to. Because there are no rules about what you do after you wake the baby up, parents can use this time to snuggle with, feed, or comfort the child as they typically would. This idea is comforting to parents who don't like the thought of causing the baby distress by taking away nighttime affection.

Drawbacks to This Approach

Because you have to be consistent about waking your baby according to a schedule, disruptions such as travel, relatives visiting, sleeping through the alarm clock, and so on can throw you off and force you to start over with the process.

It can take several weeks to completely get rid of your child's spontaneous awakenings and start to decrease the number of awakenings you control, so this is not an approach for parents who want their sleep and want it now.

It's also not an effective approach for children who have bedtime-settling problems and night-waking problems, which, to many parents' chagrin, sometimes occur in the same child.

What Parents Say About This Approach

Jill, the mother of triplets, knew she needed a method if she wanted to keep her sanity. For the first 6 weeks after her babies were born, a night nurse helped her care for the babies. Under the nurse's guidance, Jill began following a routine and eventually used the Ferber method of ignoring but checking (see Chapter 7) to teach the babies to fall asleep at night. But the babies still had night wakings—and when one baby cried, often all three would end up crying.

Jill began doing scheduled awakenings. According to a clear schedule, she would wake the babies, feed them, and put them back down to sleep.

"Night by night, we'd stretch the timing of the night feedings," she says. "By 4 months old, they were sleeping from 5 P.M. (yes—that time's right!) until 5 A.M."

She was also careful to encourage good napping during the day because she found that the better the babies slept during the day, the better they slept at night.

"I really feel lucky to have had triplets, for many reasons, but one big one is because I know I would've severely screwed up the sleep thing if I'd only had one kid at a time," she says.

The Least You Need to Know

- ◆ The "scheduled awakenings" approach can be as effective as the extinction methods (see Chapters 6, 7, and 8) but doesn't require any crying—you soothe the child as you normally would.

- ◆ Babies tend to wake at the same time every night, but by waking them ahead of time, you can eliminate the unscheduled wakings.

- ◆ Waking your child on a schedule can help him learn to sleep through the night.

- ◆ Don't let sleeping babies lie!

Chapter

11

Establishing or Changing a Bedtime Routine

In This Chapter

◆ The "bedtime routines" sleep-training approach

◆ How to get your baby into a routine so that you both can get some sleep

◆ Identifying what's not working and substituting what will

◆ Using set bedtimes and waketimes to improve your child's sleep patterns

Former senator Bob Dole once remarked after losing a campaign, "I slept like a baby. I woke up every 2 hours crying." If your baby sleeps like a baby, then maybe you need to change your routine. Even better, some experts say that establishing a routine from the start will prevent such problems from ever happening.

We'll describe how to use the "bedtime routines" approach to establish a routine that can result in a blissful night's sleep for your baby—and for you!

We'll also explain how many of the sleep problems that babies and young children experience are learned. That is, their parents "taught" them. Hey, parents get desperate and tired, and sometimes that means they reinforce bad habits. But we'll show you how to change your routine to solve the problem.

Establish or Change Your Routine

When we talk about establishing or changing your routine, we're actually talking about one of three different methods that can help your baby or child learn to fall asleep and then fall back to sleep after night wakings.

The first method is establishing a bedtime routine to signal to your child that it is time for bed. We covered this process in Chapter 8. Basically, it means having a set bedtime, a set waketime, and consistent just-before-bed habits, such as taking a bath and reading a story. This is most effective with older babies, because newborns' sleep isn't organized enough to occur on a regular schedule.

But sometimes simply establishing a regular bedtime doesn't quite solve your bedtime trials and tribulations. For example, your toddler may still resist going to bed by throwing tantrums or coming up with just one more thing she has to do before bedtime. If that's the case, you may need to do an intervention—and that means establishing "positive bedtime routines," using the method described next.

Finally, if your routine just isn't working, you may need to change it. For example, maybe your baby is used to being nursed to sleep and now needs a feeding every time she wakes up at night. Or maybe she is used to getting rocked to sleep and can't soothe herself after a night waking without your intervention. Changing the routine can fix these problems—and others like them. You need to consider what isn't working and what you can do to "change the routine" to make it work.

What It Is

Establishing *positive bedtime routines* just means you come up with some comforting bedtime rituals that help your baby realize it's bedtime, and add in a little creative scheduling to encourage your little one to fall asleep soon after his head hits the pillow.

Changing your routine means you identify what isn't working, figure out why, and substitute a more successful approach (don't worry, we'll show you how to find those more successful approaches).

> **BABY BABBLE**
>
> Establishing a **positive bedtime routine** is known in the sleep research world as "sleep hygiene." Just as you strive to keep your baby medically healthy, it's important to establish positive bedtime routines to keep his sleep healthy as well.

And in This Corner: Supporters of This Approach

Sleep researchers Drs. John Pearce and Marc Weissbluth both discuss using bedtime routines and changing the routine to solve bedtime problems. Many experts, such as Dr. Jodi Mindell, also discuss the importance of establishing a positive bedtime routine. Many agree that the "positive bedtime routine" approach is a preventative measure rather than an intervention for a problem that has already begun. But it can be used to help solve bedtime problems as well.

Creating Positive Bedtime Routines

The "bedtime routines" approach is specifically designed to avoid or solve sleep-onset problems, like tantrums, at bedtime. It's not specifically meant for night-waking problems.

However, once you deal with the sleep-onset issues, many of the night-waking problems—if your baby or child has them—will disappear, because you have taught her to self-soothe at the beginning of the night.

Positive Bedtime Routines

Here's how the "positive bedtime routines" approach works:

♦ First, decide on a goal bedtime—the time you'd like your child to consistently go to bed without difficulty each night. For example, you might choose 8 P.M. as the target bedtime.

♦ Second, move your child's bedtime *later* in the evening to better match the time that the child is currently naturally falling asleep. This will help assure that the child falls asleep soon after being put to bed.

♦ Third, establish a positive bedtime routine by choosing enjoyable bedtime activities to do together (beyond brushing teeth).

♦ Fourth, offer praise and encouragement after each activity (such as reading a story). This praise serves as a signal to your child that it's time to move on to the next activity—and eventually to bed.

♦ Finally, once this series of events has been established—a positive routine and quick sleep onset at bedtime—parents move the bedtime earlier until reaching the pre-established bedtime goal.

 Infant Almanac

Moving the bedtime earlier works best if done in 5- or 10-minute increments until your child is consistently going to bed at the goal bedtime.

Melissa's Mindset

Research shows that the "bedtime routines" approach actually produces more rapid results than Ferber's "ignore but check" method (see Chapter 7).

What you're basically doing is creating a minor degree of sleep deprivation in your child by making bedtime later. He is more likely to fall asleep quickly because he is more tired than usual. You then add in some positive bedtime routines and praise him for participating in them—relaxing activities, not a wild rumpus. This makes him feel good about bedtime. Ultimately he learns that going to sleep is a good thing. And the bedtime struggles and tantrums are over.

Changing Your Routine

The first step is admitting you have a problem ....

Once you've decided that your baby's sleep habits at bedtime *are* a problem for you and/or your baby, then you can identify what isn't working in your present routine, fix it, and create a better routine. For example ...

> **Infant Almanac**
>
> If your baby's sleep habits don't bother you and the baby is getting enough sleep, there's nothing to solve—even if your routine isn't like any of the methods described in this book.

- ◆ If you've tried the "positive bedtime routines" approach and still have trouble getting your little one to sleep at bedtime, you may need to change the activities that you do at bedtime in order to make sleep more appealing.

  - ◆ If your little one is going to sleep fine but can't seem to self-soothe after night waking, changing how you respond (e.g., changing the routine) can make all the difference.

First, identify what isn't working. Is the baby falling asleep fine at bedtime but waking an hour later? Or is your toddler resisting bedtime no matter what you seem to do? Or does your baby fall asleep only if you rock her for an hour and a half—and you'd like to have that hour and a half back?

Keep a journal of what's happening at bedtime and during the night. You want objective information that can help you figure out what to change to correct the problem. In addition, make notes about how you feel about what's happening. This subjective information is just as important: it helps you separate the annoying from the disastrous—and the disastrous problem is the one you work on first.

Maintain the sleep journal for a week or two before making any changes. Then keep track of how those changes work so that you can modify them if needed.

Bedtime Routine Daily Sleep Journal

Child's Name_____ Date_____

Bedtime Routine	What time?	How did it go?
Bath		
Clothing/diaper change		
Story		
Other pleasant activity		
Bedtime		
Night wakings		
First		
Second		
Third		

Infant Almanac

If you feel that your method isn't working but aren't sure what steps to take, talk to your pediatrician about options. Better yet, find a pediatric sleep center and talk to a doctor who has been trained specifically in the area of sleep. Many pediatricians do not receive training related to sleep and may not be prepared to accurately dispense sleep advice. See Appendix B for more information about pediatric sleep centers.

Possible Problems

Look at your bedtime routines and consider how you may be contributing to your baby's sleep difficulty.

Problem #1: If you put your baby to bed only after she has already fallen asleep, she is likely to need your help to fall asleep again when she wakes during the night.

Solution: Change your routine by putting the baby to bed when she is awake, at least sometimes. Drowsy is ideal; half-asleep is fine; barely conscious is acceptable. But she can't be snoozing away or you'll just reinforce a bad habit.

Problem #2: If you check on your baby each time he makes a sound at night, he may require your presence to fall back asleep.

Solution: Sometimes your presence actually rouses the baby further. He might be able to go back to sleep without any help if you let him try. Make sure he's really awake before going to him.

Problem #3: Your baby goes to bed fine but wakes up an hour later needing to be fed.

Solution: Try giving your baby a full feeding before bedtime; then wake the baby up before you go to bed and try another feeding.

Problem #4: Your baby is used to nursing herself to sleep.

Solution: Try changing the routine to massaging your baby, cuddling her, or singing her a lullaby (or any combination of these). Anything to change the association that nursing equals sleep.

Problem #5: Your baby resists going back to sleep without a feeding if mother goes to comfort him.

Solution: Try having father (or another adult) put the baby to sleep.

Perhaps your problem is different or more persistent. Consider these questions:

- ◆ Are you a good sleep role model? Do you get enough sleep? What are your bedtime routines and habits? Can you improve them?

- ◆ Who is involved in your child's bedtime routine? Could it be changed or modified?

- ◆ Are you consistent in other areas of your child's life? Or do you need to be more consistent with "yes" and "no" during the day to reinforce what you're trying to do at night?

- ◆ Does your partner agree with your sleep routine?

- ◆ If your partner thinks you should try a different bedtime routine, have you tried it?

- ◆ Do you reward an older child if he rested well and stayed in bed?

◆ Is there stress in your family that could be affecting your child's sleep habits? What can you do about it?

◆ Have you let someone besides you or your partner put your baby to bed? For example, a sitter or grandmother? What happened?

◆ Have you consulted a sleep professional?

Challenges You'll Encounter

Identifying what the problem is and finding a successful solution for it is the biggest challenge with this approach, because you run the risk of trading one problem for another.

Also, you may second-guess yourself and not give the change in routine enough time to work effectively. And it's easy to fall back into the same habits even if you've decided that you want to take a different approach.

Advantages to Establishing or Changing the Routine Approaches

The definition of insanity is doing the same thing over and over again and expecting different results. With the "change the routine" approach, you're given free rein to make changes that will produce different (and one hopes more positive) results—and less insanity.

Creating positive bedtime routines prevents long bouts of crying and reduced anxiety on your part, and can head off sleep problems before they start.

Drawbacks to Establishing or Changing the Routine Approaches

The main drawback to changing the routine is that there's no way of knowing whether your routine change is going to work. This makes it harder to stay committed to changing poor sleep habits.

Creating positive bedtime routines requires a time commitment and can be disrupted by travel or illness.

What Parents Say About This Approach

Debbie used both the "bedtime routines" and the "changing the routine" approaches. She says that her daughter would cry whenever Debbie and her husband put her down for bedtime. So they tried changing their routine a few different ways: "We tried swinging the baby, rocking the baby, nursing the baby to sleep, playing 'white' noise, you name it. We knew we were supposed to put her down awake so she could learn to sleep on her own, but we were so desperate we tried putting her down asleep. That didn't work either—she awoke the second she was in the crib."

Then they regrouped and developed a different bedtime routine for their daughter and kept to it even though she did cry a little when she was put down for bedtime. It took a few weeks, but now "she and our son, with whom we used the same method, are extremely easy to get to sleep. Our family, babysitters, and friends marvel at how we go through our bedtime routine (which includes one story and one song after teeth brushing) and then we kiss them goodnight and shut the door. Rarely a peep."

The Least You Need to Know

- ◆ Creating a positive bedtime routine can help your child develop good sleep habits, enabling everyone to get a good night's sleep.
- ◆ If it's broke, fix it.
- ◆ Changing the routine can correct poor sleep habits in your baby.
- ◆ Creative problem-solving helps you and your baby get a good night's rest.

Chapter 12

Sharing the Bed

In This Chapter

- ◆ The "co-sleeping" sleep-training approach
- ◆ Benefits of attachment parenting
- ◆ How co-sleeping can help you get some sleep
- ◆ Keeping the family bed safe and secure

In this chapter, we'll show you how the family that sleeps together ... er ... gets some sleep. We'll discuss how to set up a family bed so that your baby will be safe and secure, and we'll discuss potential safety concerns and how to address them. We'll also show you how the family bed doesn't have to mean the end of your love life, and we'll describe how you can eventually transition your child to a room (and a bed) of his own.

The "Co-Sleeping" Approach

Co-sleeping means simply having your baby sleep in the same bed as you do. The family bed can expand to include both parents, their other children, and their new baby.

BABY BABBLE

Co-sleeping means sharing your bed with your baby. It goes by many other names: the family bed, bed-sharing, sleep-sharing.

Melissa's Mindset

Technically, "co-sleeping" is the term used to describe a shared sleeping space, which may or may not involve sleeping in the same bed. Researchers use the terms "bed-sharing" and "room-sharing" to be more specific. For the purpose of this chapter, the term "co-sleeping" will be used to refer to sleeping in the same bed.

We do need to tell you, though, that in 2005, the American Academy of Pediatrics came out with a controversial statement cautioning against bed-sharing because of a few reports of parents rolling over on their babies in bed. One study that suggests co-sleeping on sofas is a risk factor for Sudden Infant Death Syndrome (SIDS). The AAP now recommends room-sharing for the first year, but not co-sleeping. Bear this in mind as you make your decision.

Many in the sleep community feel the statement goes too far, as many cultures do sleep with their babies safely. There is no indication that safe co-sleeping is related to any deaths and, in fact, many supporters of co-sleeping contend that co-sleeping babies are less likely to suffer SIDS or other life-threatening medical conditions, because parents are right there to handle emergencies.

What It Is

Co-sleeping is a way for parents and babies to bond and for each to get more sleep. People who want to do *attachment parenting* often co-sleep, but not all co-sleepers are supporters of the "attachment-parenting" approach.

Dr. William Sears, one of the best-known supporters of attachment parenting (not to mention co-sleeping), lists "the seven Bs" of attachment parenting:

- ◆ Birth-bonding (holding and touching your newborn immediately after birth)
- ◆ Breastfeeding

- Baby-wearing (using slings to keep baby next to you as much as possible)

- Bed-sharing

- Belief in baby's cries (responding to crying as communication, not manipulation)

- Balance and boundaries

- Beware of baby trainers—experts who will tell you how to care for your baby without ever meeting your baby!

> **B A B Y   B A B B L E**
>
> **Attachment parenting** is simply letting your baby guide you in your decision making.

Attachment-parenting babies, according to Sears, are smarter, healthier, and better behaved than their peers.

Time for another disclaimer. In this chapter, we discuss "proactive" co-sleeping, which is when parents plan and enjoy the practice of bed-sharing. But sometimes parents react to sleep problems in their children and end up sharing the same bed out of desperation. "Reactive" co-sleeping is considered more problematic by some sleep clinicians, who see reactive co-sleeping as an indication of a sleep disorder in the child.

Melissa's Mindset

There is no research to support Dr. Sears' claim that these babies are smarter, healthier, or better behaved than their solitary-sleeping counterparts. For some babies and parents, this is a healthy approach to nighttime sleep, but it is not a recipe for creating a Superchild. (If only!)

There is no evidence that *proactive* co-sleeping is associated with sleep problems, and, in fact, the connection between reactive co-sleeping and sleep problems is not clear—the problem probably existed before the co-sleeping did.

In a nutshell? If you choose this approach, be sure you're doing it in a conscious, planned, and thoughtful way, and not just in reaction to sleep problems that your child is experiencing.

And in This Corner: Supporters of This Approach

Dr. Williams Sears, one of the main proponents of attachment parenting, is one of the best-known supporters of the family bed. He talks about this approach in *Nighttime Parenting* and *The Baby Sleep Book*, two of several books published with his wife, Martha.

Jay Gordon, M.D. and Maria Goodavage write about successfully sharing the family bed in their book, *Good Nights*.

Using This Approach

Babies are supposed to sleep with parents, say supporters of this approach. It's only natural. Human touch is necessary to your baby's survival, and the family bed is one way to ensure that your baby gets enough of it. Babies sleep better, cry less, and grow faster with plenty of touch, and they find it extremely stressful to be separated from parents.

> **Infant Almanac**
>
> According to family bed supporters, near contact (preferably skin to skin) with parents helps the baby regulate vital functions such as heart rate, hormone levels, blood pressure, and body temperature.

> **Melissa's Mindset**
>
> It makes sense that back in the caveman days, babies must have co-slept in order to avoid being snatched by saber-tooth tigers and such. Supporters of co-sleeping cite the fact that the majority of cultures in the world still do sleep with their babies nearby. Some parents in different cultures find the Western practice of independent sleep barbaric and cruel.

The family bed has many benefits:

♦ Breastfeeding goes naturally with the family bed, reinforcing the healthiest nutritional option of breastfeeding your infant.

♦ You can also use the family bed if you're bottle-feeding, by keeping the bottles and warmer at bedside.

♦ It's safer than solitary sleeping, say supporters (who point out that the Sudden Infant Death Syndrome rates are highest in industrial societies where infants sleep separately from their parents).

♦ Babies cry less because parents are right there to comfort them.

♦ Babies grow into well-adjusted children and adults.

♦ Mothers experience longer, more refreshing sleep periods when co-sleeping.

- Fathers are able to participate more, by helping soothe baby back to sleep.

- Parents of multiples are not as sleep deprived.

- Parents are able to immediately help a child in trouble from choking, sleep apnea (breathing cessation), and other medical problems.

- Parents can immediately help their child in nonmedical emergencies, such as a fire.

- Babies don't rely on transitional objects and pacifiers. Instead they learn to rely on people to help them.

- Parents can still have an active, er, you know—the thing that brought you the baby in the first place—although they may have to get a little inventive about making it happen (see "Getting a Little Lovin'," following).

Melissa's Mindset

Again, there is no research-based evidence to support any of these claims. It is unlikely that the family bed or solitary sleeping directly cause any behavioral or emotional issues. There are more important factors involved, such as a child's temperament, her genes, and the quality of her environment that are more likely to strongly impact her development than the experience of shared or independent sleep.

At the same time, according to family-bed supporters, children who don't benefit from the family bed are harder to control, are unhappier, more stressed, more fearful, more prone to peer pressure, and develop more behavior and emotional problems for which they seek help. Whew!

Step-by-Step

The most important "rule" of the family bed is to keep it safe, so the first step is to establish a family agreement concerning how you'll sleep with the baby.

You'll want to use the following guidelines as a place to start your "safety first" campaign:

- No smoking. Smoking increases the risk of SIDS and endangers a baby in the family bed.

Unhappy Baby Alert

The family bed requires everyone involved to be committed to it. So if one parent is against it, it will not be successful. And parents must be committed to safety and sobriety to ensure the baby's safety. If this is not possible, another approach should be used.

♦ Don't co-sleep when under the influence of illicit drugs, alcohol, or any substance that may affect your ability to sense and respond to your baby.

♦ Don't co-sleep if you're overly exhausted—you're more likely to accidentally "overlie" (roll over on) your baby and not realize it.

♦ Use a firm mattress only and make sure the bed frame fits snugly against the mattress.

♦ Avoid headboards and footboards that have rails or slots where the baby could trap his head.

♦ The bigger the bed, the safer everyone in it is.

♦ Obese adults are less aware of the baby's proximity to their bodies and must exercise additional care or consider not co-sleeping.

♦ Don't place the bed against a wall. This is one way that babies get trapped.

♦ Keep the bed low to the ground. One alternative is to place the mattress directly on the floor.

♦ Use thin blankets, not quilts or down comforters, to prevent possible suffocation.

 Melissa's Mindset

While nothing is risk free, you can reduce the risk of the family bed by understanding the hazards—the baby getting trapped or wedged between the mattress and other objects (such as a wall), suffocating in a water bed or downy comforter, or strangling in rails and other openings.

♦ Don't allow pillows near the baby (same reason).

♦ Ban the fluffy stuffed animals (ditto).

♦ Put the baby to sleep on her back.

♦ Keep long hair pulled back.

♦ Childproof your bedroom (he'll be climbing out of bed on his own before you know it).

Where to position the baby on the bed depends on who else is in the bed. If other children are in the family bed, keep an adult between the infant and the child. Children are not as aware of the baby as adults are. Make sure the baby sleeps by Mom if Dad sleeps very soundly. Mothers are more likely to be aware of the baby's proximity.

Melissa's Mindset

Consider using a crib-type bed that attaches to your bed. The baby sleeps next to you but is less vulnerable to overlying, wedging, and other dangers. In addition to a side-car-style bassinet that attaches to the bed, a mini-bassinet now on the market can be placed on the mattress. It has small sides that keep the baby separate from parents and prevent overlying.

Step Two

Wait, there is no step two. Once you've organized the family bed safely, the process is simple. No complicated bedtime routine is needed, although you can establish one if you wish. Simply let the baby fall asleep with you in bed.

If it's not your bedtime, you can get up once the baby is deeply asleep. For a young baby, this might take 20 to 30 minutes; for an older baby, 10 minutes.

Naps are a little different from bedtime because it's not safe to allow the baby to nap alone on the bed. You can always put your baby to nap in the crib that would otherwise collect dust. If you'd rather not (or you don't even have a crib), try the following:

Infant Almanac

One of the benefits of co-sleeping is that everyone in the bed begins to synchronize their sleep. So they're all deeply asleep at the same time and more lightly asleep at the same time. Thus, night wakings aren't as much trouble and disruptive.

♦ Use guardrails on your bed to prevent the baby from rolling off.

♦ Wear the baby in a sling while she naps.

♦ Use a baby swing for naps.

Night Wakings

Even though you're co-sleeping with your baby, you'll probably have as many night wakings as any other parent. (We're sorry to have to break the news to you.)

Here's how to deal with night wakings:

♦ If the baby needs to be fed, often she will latch on to a breastfeeding mother and both will quickly fall asleep again.

♦ A bottle-fed baby can easily be fed if equipment is near at hand; though the parent is awake longer to do the feeding, there is less disruption because no one gets out of bed, fetches the baby, spills the milk all over the floor, and so on.

> **Infant Almanac**
>
> Lots of famous parents have used the family bed: singer-songwriter Kenny Loggins, actor Pierce Brosnan, writer Maya Angelou. You're in good company!

♦ If the baby just wants to play at night, ignore him.

♦ Keep the nighttime quiet and calm.

Getting a Little Lovin'

Critics of the family bed say it puts a damper on your love life and may actually hide problems you're having with your spouse. Nonsense, say supporters. In fact, they say the family bed can improve your love life. Consider the following:

♦ Most co-sleeping parents don't do it in the family bed, so no one's going to get warped from the experience. Parents just get inventive.

♦ The intimacy of the family bed increases the love and compassion between the parents.

♦ It requires planning and ingenuity to get a little action, which can make it more fun and exciting.

♦ The family bed enables you to get enough sleep to actually have a libido.

- Making time for each other will benefit your relationship in other ways.

- Making dates with each other will also benefit your relationship.

Moving Beyond the Family Bed

Eventually you're going to have to move your child out of your bed (presumably sometime before college). This can be easy or hard, depending on the child:

- The child may decide himself that he's ready for his own bed. Children are often around 4 years old when they reach this conclusion.

- A new baby will usually help the older sibling move to her own bed, though we don't recommend getting pregnant just to get your bed back.

- A gentle transition can be accomplished to encourage your child to accept his own bed.

How to go about creating this gentle transition?

- Talk to the child about being in her own bed eventually.

- Create a space or room of the child's own.

- Put him in a bed of his own in your room.

- Move her into a room with an older sibling.

- Let the child fall asleep in your bed, and then move to her own bed.

- Put the child to bed in his own room but allow him to come to your bed if needed after waking at night.

Challenges You'll Encounter

It can be difficult to fall asleep if you're afraid of rolling over onto the baby!

The family bed may do nothing to reduce the number of night wakings a baby has (although they will be less disruptive because the baby is likely to cry less with you right there).

Coping with naysayers can also be difficult. Without the right support and information, you may give up when your mother-in-law says your kids are going to turn into spoiled, clingy monsters.

Advantages to This Approach

Ninety-eight percent of the 250 parents Dr. Gordon interviewed for his book *Good Nights* would do it again, so they must be doing something right!

Parents report feeling more intimate and loving, not just to the baby but to each other. Many report less-disrupted sleep and a much easier time breastfeeding. From the baby's point of view, there's a lot less crying.

Drawbacks to This Approach

If everyone involved is not equally committed, it can be hard to work through the challenges. Also, if one person doesn't take the safety issues seriously enough, the approach should not be used.

Melissa's Mindset

Keep in mind that some babies simply don't like to sleep with others. I've known plenty of families who planned to co-sleep but ended up not doing so because the baby slept better independently. Flexibility is key.

It can be difficult to wean the child from the family bed. While some children naturally decide they want to move into their own bed—sometimes in the same room, and eventually into a room of their own—not all children are so inclined and you may have to push them to do so.

What Parents Say About This Approach

For Melissa, co-sleeping was a natural urge that began immediately after she gave birth to Nickolas. She wanted to have him close during sleep, and he did sleep for longer periods of time when co-sleeping. The day she brought Nickolas home from the hospital, she had set up a bassinet right next to the bed, thinking that he would sleep there. But, that first night, she realized that even the bassinet was too far away for the tiny guy. Nick would squirm and reach out, never seeming to get comfortable. When she slept with him, both of them settled in and slept better. It made nighttime nursing much easier as well.

Melissa continued to sleep with Nick for the first few months of his life. He slept during the day in a crib or bassinet, but nighttimes were spent together. This was important for Melissa, because she went back to work immediately after giving birth. The nighttime snuggles helped to establish their relationship and gave them special time together that they did not have during the day.

It was a humbling experience, because Melissa had originally thought that co-sleeping was a weird alternative practice and had been skeptical about it from her first introduction to co-sleeping families in graduate school. This attitude clearly changed once she had her own child.

Yes, Melissa had to deal with well-meaning family and friends who thought the practice was weird or would lead to a dependent child. But she was able to discuss research showing that this was not true, so the naysayers eventually left it alone. Nickolas is now a well-adjusted 4-year-old, and the two still find co-sleeping an enjoyable time to be together … for at least part of the night. This approach was a good match for them.

The Least You Need to Know

- The family bed can be a safe, nurturing space for your baby.
- Co-sleeping can encourage bonding with all family members.
- Co-sleeping requires careful attention to safety issues.
- Yes, you can get a little lovin' despite sharing your bed with the new baby. You just have to be creative!

Chapter 13

The Tear-Free Zone

In This Chapter

- The "persistent gentle removal system" sleep-training approach
- Striking a balance between "cry it out" and "live with it"
- Creating a sleep plan based on your baby
- Making the right sleep associations for your baby

Many parents are philosophically opposed to "cry it out" approaches—or else they tried one and couldn't bear it—but they don't realize there are "tear-free" or "mostly tear-free" approaches they can try—sleep training methods that don't demand that you let your baby cry it out.

The "persistent gentle removal system" is supposed to help you strike a balance between letting your baby cry it out and just living with your baby's sleep problems.

The "Persistent Gentle Removal System" Approach

BABY BABBLE

Sleep associations are objects and activities that your baby connects with falling asleep.

Infant Almanac

You can use the "persistent gentle removal system" approach with co-sleeping and breastfeeding or with any other choice you might make.

This approach is used to eliminate night wakings by changing the *sleep associations* your infant has. For example, babies who are rocked to sleep have trouble soothing themselves from night wakings without parental intervention, so this approach will require you to change your ways.

What It Is

This approach requires you to create a daily routine and to make positive sleep associations—those being activities and objects that the baby identifies with sleep but which you don't have to be present to do. For example, a positive sleep association might be to put the baby to sleep in a dark, quiet room. You don't have to be in the room for it to be dark and quiet—you just keep the lights off and the cat out.

In addition, you use a sleep log to identify your baby's pattern and learn how to adapt to it (or change it, if needed).

And in This Corner: Supporters of This Approach

Elizabeth Pantley, mother of four and a parent educator, writes about this approach in her book, *The No-Cry Sleep Solution*. Tammy Hussin, a mother of three, advocates a similar approach in her book, *Sleep Baby Sleep*. (Hussin's book is not a researched approach and relies heavily on anecdotal information.)

Using This Approach

Using the "gentle" approach, you'll educate yourself about the amount of sleep your baby needs and what to expect as far as night wakings.

With this information, you're better prepared to cope with your baby and her needs. You'll also establish and maintain a regular schedule to help keep your baby from getting overtired and to help her learn good sleep habits.

Step-by-Step

Begin by keeping a sleep log so you can recognize your baby's habits and patterns and then gradually change those sleep associations. This way, you don't always have to be there for your baby to fall asleep at bedtime and to go back to sleep after a night waking. Then you'll track the baby's night wakings on a separate log (this one has slightly different categories). Adapt the logs as appropriate.

> **Infant Almanac**
>
> Remember, "sleeping through the night" is generally considered 5 hours, such as from midnight to 5 A.M. Most parents don't consider that a full night's sleep.

Sleep Associations Daily Sleep Log

Date: _____ Nap _____ or Bedtime _____

Time you began morning nap ritual

What you were doing_____

The environment:

    Activity level _____

    Noise _____

    Lighting _____

Time baby fell asleep _____

How baby fell asleep
(rocking, nursing) _____

Where baby fell asleep
(in crib, in mother's arms) _____

Length of sleep_____

Time you began afternoon nap ritual

What you were doing_____

The environment:
    Activity level _____

    Noise _____

    Lighting_____

Time baby fell asleep _____

How baby fell asleep
(rocking, nursing) _____

Where baby fell asleep
(in crib, in mother's arms) _____

Length of sleep _____

Time you began bedtime ritual

What you were doing _____

The environment:
    Activity level _____

    Noise _____

    Lighting_____

Time baby fell asleep _____

How baby fell asleep
(rocking, nursing) _____

Where baby fell asleep
(in crib, in mother's arms) _____

Length of sleep _____

Sleep Associations Night Wakings Log

Date: _____

Night waking #1

Time baby awoke _____

Wake signal (cry, movement)_____

Length of waketime _____

What you did_____

Time baby went back to sleep _____

Night waking #2

Time baby awoke _____

Wake signal (cry, movement)_____

Length of waketime _____

What you did_____

Time baby went back to sleep _____

Night waking #3

Time baby awoke _____

Wake signal (cry, movement)_____

Length of waketime _____

What you did_____

Time baby went back to sleep _____

From this information, you can create a plan to help encourage the child to go to sleep at bedtime without too much fuss and to go back to sleep after a night waking. Here are some examples:

- If your baby is having fewer naps than needed, you can encourage more.

- If a more consistent bedtime is needed, you can stick more strictly to a schedule.

- If you have a haphazard bedtime routine, you can create a more reliable one.

According to supporters of this approach, methods you'll use to help your baby sleep through the night include the following:

- When the baby is asleep for a nap, put him to sleep in his own bed (even if co-sleeping—adults don't need as much sleep as babies and you shouldn't have to be there all the time).

- Don't let baby always fall asleep while rocking or nursing or she won't be able to fall asleep any other way.

- Put the baby to bed drowsy, not asleep, when possible.

- If he doesn't fall asleep, pat, rock, pick him up, feed him—do whatever you need to do. There's no need for him to cry it out.

Creating a Routine Schedule

Infant Almanac

Sleeping in on the weekends may seem like a good way to overcome your sleep deprivation, but it can disrupt your baby. Oversleeping on the weekends actually may be a sign that you are sleep- deprived, and can disrupt your natural circadian rhythms. Instead, try to get an adequate amount of sleep during the entire week.

You need to have a fairly routine schedule during both days and nights for your baby to eventually adjust and learn to sleep through the night. This includes setting ...

- Regular mealtimes.

- Regular play times.

- Regular naps.

- A predictable routine: each morning you wake at the same time, get dressed, have breakfast, play.

Planning for Night Wakings

Most important, accept that your baby will wake at night. Plan for those wakings by doing the following:

- Keep what you need in an easily accessible place.

- Place a comfortable chair in the nursery.

- Use nursing pillows and other props to prevent strains.

- Arrange your schedule around the baby for the first few months.

- Take a break! It's okay to slow down now.

Creating Positive Sleep Associations

Your baby associates certain objects and activities with sleep. The more you can encourage these associations to not include you, the more likely your baby will learn to fall asleep on her own and go back to sleep after a night waking.

Some of these strategies may help:

◆ Make the bed seem like a good place to hang out. Put baby in the crib with a toy while you sit nearby. The idea is to get your baby to have positive feelings while in the crib.

◆ Use different methods to help baby fall asleep so that she doesn't associate any one method with falling asleep. Try a swing, car ride, rocking, singing, nursing.

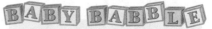

> A **lovey** is a transitional object—a favorite toy or blanket the comforts the baby. Most babies don't choose a consistent lovey until after the first year of life, but many use a variety of different things (pacifiers, blankets, toys) during the first year.

◆ Encourage the use of a *"lovey,"* such as a favorite toy or blanket. (Very young babies do not get attached to loveys, so this is a strategy for the older baby.)

◆ Develop sound cues—words you use or music you play that indicates bedtime.

Encouraging the Tired Newborn to Sleep

Often, babies have trouble sleeping not because they aren't tired but because they *are* tired—they're too tired to sleep.

Advocates of this approach suggest trying some of these methods of positive sleep associations to get your little one to go nighty-night:

◆ Swaddle your baby.

◆ Use a smaller crib or bassinet.

◆ Allow your baby to sleep in a car seat or stroller.

Infant Almanac

> To help your baby distinguish night from day, let her take naps in more brightly lit areas but put her to bed in a dark, quiet room.

Melissa's Mindset

Many developmentalists oppose allowing babies to sleep in car seats, strollers, or swings for extended periods of time. Extensive use of these devices has been associated with "deformational plagiocephaly" (say that 10 times fast!). This is basically a permanently misshapen head.

◆ Use a sling—a cloth baby holder to keep your child close to your body but enabling you to use your hands.

◆ Warm the bed with an electric blanket or hot water bottle before putting baby down (take the blanket or bottle away before putting baby down).

◆ Put on soft music or white noise.

Needy Nursers

Some babies nurse very frequently or need to suck a pacifier to soothe themselves. For these babies, try the following steps:

1. When baby wakes, give her a pacifier or nurse her.

2. Don't leave baby with a pacifier in her mouth or let her fall asleep with it in her mouth.

3. After allowing her to suck for a few minutes, remove the breast/bottle or pacifier.

Infant Almanac

The American Academy of Pediatrics now recommends nighttime pacifier use for babies. They say babies should be encouraged to use a pacifier at bedtime through the first year of life.

4. If baby objects, continue to allow pacifier or breast/bottle.

5. Remove pacifier or breast/bottle before baby falls asleep.

6. Repeat every night as needed.

7. Baby will eventually learn (usually before college) to sleep without nursing or needing a pacifier.

Challenges You'll Encounter

It's easy to fall into old habits (letting your baby fall asleep before putting him down for a nap), especially when they work.

Sleep-deprived parents may not want to deal with the paperwork of logging their baby's sleep habits.

This system is probably most applicable for babies who are easy sleepers to begin with. For children with established sleep problems, this gentle, unstructured approach may actually make the problem worse.

Advantages to This Approach

This system is, indeed, gentle. You don't have to feel like a terrible parent for letting your child cry it out because your child doesn't cry it out.

The baby eventually learns to fall asleep on his own but does not lose trust in you, and knows that you will be there to comfort him.

Drawbacks to This Approach

It may take a long time (thus the word "persistent" in the name) for this method to work, so parents need to be dedicated and committed.

This approach may be too gentle for some babies who won't get the hint. Some parents may want to see results sooner rather than later. Many experts would say that, because this approach allows parents to do what they want if the baby gets upset, the sleep problem could potentially worsen.

Melissa's Mindset

There is no research on this approach, and no indication that using different methods to get the baby to sleep at night will teach the baby to fall asleep on her own.

What Parents Say About This Approach

While supporters of this approach share anecdotal evidence that it can work, we weren't able to find any parents who had tried it and had success. Melissa also looked at the research and could not find case histories that would indicate that this method is effective. In fact, Melissa expresses concern that this method could reinforce sleep problems, especially since intermittent reinforcement is the best way to ensure that a certain behavior continues. For example, if a baby consistently nurses to sleep and you try to take away that association, the baby will cry. If you then continue to nurse, that would only reinforce the crying every time you try to stop nursing.

The Least You Need to Know

♦ Your baby can learn to fall asleep by himself without crying it out.

♦ Changing your baby's sleep associations can help her learn to fall asleep and go back to sleep after a night waking.

♦ Creating a predictable routine throughout the day and night will help your baby develop good sleep habits.

♦ Planning for night wakings instead of hoping they'll go away will help you handle them better.

Chapter

14

Letting the Child Outgrow It

In This Chapter

- ◆ The "wait it out" approach
- ◆ Using patience instead of training to help your child learn to sleep
- ◆ When waiting it out can be an effective strategy for your baby or child's sleep problem
- ◆ Tossing out schedules and letting your baby lead the way

"Patience is a virtue, possess it if you can." That old cliché will never seem truer if you decide to simply wait out your baby's or child's sleep problems. But while you may wear your patience thin, your baby won't be shedding too many tears. Instead, he'll learn that he can rely on you to take care of business ... business as usual, that is.

In this chapter, we'll show how using the "wait it out" approach can help you deal with sleep issues—without resorting to strict schedules, ignoring it, and other methods that may seem a little too cold and unkind for your baby. But although some sleep problems can be solved with patience, others require direct intervention. That's why we'll give you some information on how to decide which category your baby's or child's sleep problem falls into.

The "Wait It Out" Approach

Just as it sounds, the "wait it out" approach means that you and the rest of the family hunker down and put up with some nighttime challenges, hoping that your baby will outgrow her problems and eventually organize her sleep so that everyone can get a little shut-eye.

Even if you intend to use a stricter method of sleep training later on, you should realize that it is not appropriate to try to change the sleep patterns of very young infants. Young babies should be waking up at night; it actually may be problematic for them to sleep through the night, due to Sudden Infant Death Syndrome (SIDS) concerns. It will be necessary to wait until the baby is developmentally ready to sleep for longer stretches of time.

Melissa's Mindset

Most experts agree that strict sleep training should not be used with infants until after 3–6 months of age. However, during the first few months, parents can try to establish good sleep habits to prevent problems from occurring in the first place.

In addition, there may be certain reasons, owing to emotional or physical problems, when sleep training would not be a good idea for your baby or child. See Chapter 4 for more information about this.

What It Is

Using the "wait it out" approach, you don't train your baby by ignoring her. You don't, in fact, use any particular method to train your baby to fall asleep by herself and to go back to sleep after a night waking. You respond to the baby as needed, and do whatever it takes to comfort her.

If you think this sounds is similar to the "persistent gentle removal system" approach described in Chapter 13, you're right. Only in this case you're not trying to change sleep associations, you're just trying to give the baby a little time and space to figure things out on her own.

And in This Corner: Supporters of This Approach

Some physicians are indirectly supporters of this approach, since they feel that babies will outgrow most sleep problems eventually and that, in any case, such problems aren't in any sense disorders that need to be treated. Eventually the baby will figure out how to sleep on his own.

Advocates of co-sleeping (see Chapter 12) often encourage a "wait it out" approach, saying that the child will eventually transition to her own bed and sleep through the night without much in the way of parental training or intervention, if she is allowed to take the lead and if parents follow her cues.

It's important to remember that not all co-sleepers elect to co-sleep out of a reaction to the baby's sleep problems. Some co-sleeping families do so out of preference and do not consider co-sleeping either a sign or a symptom of a sleep problem. See Chapter 12 for more information on co-sleeping.

Using This Approach

Some sleep problems are eventually outgrown, say advocates of this approach. Sometimes problems are transient and may be due to developmental transitions. For example, some research has shown that when babies are first learning to walk, their sleep becomes disrupted for a short period of time. Once their brains have acclimated to the new physical activity, they experience better sleep.

Unhappy Baby Alert

If you choose the "wait it out" approach, make sure that you take care of yourself, too. Going in to comfort a baby three times a night is wearing. If you're sleep deprived and miserable, you'll pass that along to your baby—resulting in an unhappy baby. So be sure to get the help you need, take breaks when you can, and don't overextend yourself.

Melissa's Mindset

Most sleep clinicians report that night-waking or sleep-onset problems that continue after the first year of life should not be ignored. Sleep specialists say that sleep problems tend to persist, and may either get worse or change into a different kind of sleep problem with time. If parents are concerned with their child's sleep, they should see a sleep specialist rather than wait it out.

Newborns aren't capable of sleeping through the night, but eventually they mature enough so that they can. Those difficulties that plague toddler and school-age children, like bedwetting, nightmares, and night terrors, are also usually outgrown without medical or parental intervention. (See Chapters 16 and 17 for more information about these sleep disruptions.)

Thus, waiting for the child to grow up a little is a sensible solution to many nighttime problems.

Melissa's Mindset

There is some research that supports the idea that babies will outgrow sleeping difficulties. Most studies include what is known as a "control group" when they are comparing different sleep-training approaches. The control group's sleep is measured in the same way as the training group's, but no method is used to try to change the control group's sleep. Studies have found that as many as 36 percent of babies stop waking up at night on their own after just 8 weeks. Another longer study found that across 5 years, babies who had been waking at night stopped doing so. The point is that sometimes just waiting it out really can work.

Step-by-Step

Infant Almanac

Supporters of the "wait it out" approach say that most sleep problems that babies and young children have aren't really problems for them—they are problems for their parents!

Instead of training your child to not need your presence or contorting yourself to alter his sleep associations, you just give him what he seems to need with the confidence that he will eventually outgrow the need for you to help him get to sleep.

If your baby likes, as Jennifer's daughter did, falling asleep in the mechanical swing, then you just keep doing that until the baby doesn't need to do it anymore. The same with driving around the block, rocking until your arms are numb, nursing on demand. The baby will let you know when she is ready to move along.

The idea behind *baby-led weaning* is that your baby will eventually wean himself or herself from needing you to perform a certain task to help him sleep.

However, you'll find it easier to wait it out if you follow these strategies:

- ◆ Keep consistent bed and wake times.

- ◆ Follow a bedtime routine.

- ◆ Maintain a cool, dark, quiet nursery.

BABY BABBLE

Baby-led weaning is relying on the baby to let you know when he or she is ready to be weaned from any activity that depends on you—nursing, co-sleeping, and so forth.

- ◆ Make the nursery/bedroom a place to sleep only.

Doing so encourages the child to get the sleep necessary for her health and development.

Just because you are taking the child's lead and waiting for her to outgrow minor sleep issues does not mean that you need to be a complete pushover. Parents should follow these strategies to make sure the child gets the sleep she needs. Otherwise, you could end up with an overtired child, or worse yet, create a persistent sleep problem that does require intervention.

Challenges You'll Encounter

The baby may eventually learn to organize his own sleep, but he may be 3 or 4 years old before this happens. Some parents simply can't put up with night wakings or bedtime challenges for that long.

In addition, some sleep problems will not go away on their own, and ignoring them will actually make them worse.

Advantages to This Approach

Fewer tears and power struggles means that you and your baby can get to know each other. You learn what your baby needs instead of trying to impose your own schedule on her.

Drawbacks to This Approach

Being able to deal with night wakings for months—even several years—can try even the most committed parent's patience.

In the same way, waiting for the baby to outgrow the need to nurse to sleep may take a long time unless the parent is willing to encourage the transition.

What Parents Say About This Approach

Diana says, "We never followed a method with our son. We knew about them all but believed that every child is different. We had the luxury of being able to do some different, creative things since both my husband and I work at home. So if he had a rough night, we didn't have to leave for work at 7 A.M."

Diana and her husband always looked to him for cues about what he needed. "We're really very loosey-goosey about sleeping," she says. "It works for us. He's always been a good sleeper—after the first 6 weeks, which were awful. He's a night owl, but that's okay with us. He has a regular waketime, and we remind him of that now that he's old enough to understand." Her son is now 4.

Diana and her husband co-slept with their son at first. Then he decided to transition to his own room. "Now he has a nest in his father's office. He'll fall asleep there and Dad will bring him to his room. He can come to our bed if he wants, but generally he does stay in bed all night." This relaxed approach means that Diana has never experienced sleep problems the way other parents do. Bad nights happen occasionally as they do for any parent, but letting her son outgrow—or grow into—each stage has resulted in less stress all around.

The Least You Need to Know

♦ Some say that most babies and children learn to sleep through the night no matter what you do—or don't do.

♦ Waiting it out can be an appealing alternative if you don't want to listen to your baby cry it out.

♦ Letting your child outgrow sleep problems requires patience.

♦ You can use this approach while also creating daily schedules and a nightly bedtime ritual to encourage your child to fall asleep and go back to sleep after night wakings.

Chapter 15

Combining Sleep-Training Approaches

In This Chapter

- Why combining sleep-training approaches might be right for you and your baby
- How the sleep experts combine approaches
- Choosing compatible sleep-training approaches
- Avoiding setbacks when combining approaches
- Identifying when and why to combine approaches

A pinch of this, a smidgen of that, and you have the recipe for a good night's sleep … or else an unmitigated disaster. How do you improve your chances for getting the good night's sleep instead of the unmitigated disaster? By combining approaches with care.

Combining sleep-training approaches is a tactic that sleep experts use to help their patients get some shut-eye. If you think about it, using a couple of sleep-training methods may seem like choosing the best of all possible worlds—but it goes without saying that you have to be smart about how you do it or you'll end up undermining your own efforts.

Melissa's Mindset

Many sleep experts recommend that sleep-training techniques be adapted to better fit individual families' and infants' needs. This means that combined approaches are often used when treating sleep problems.

In this chapter, we'll show you why you might consider combining approaches, and how you can choose compatible approaches to mix. We'll give you hints for making the most of the methods and working with them to create an approach that will be just right for you and your baby. And we'll describe why sleep experts do just this to help their patients with their sleep problems.

The Combined Approach

Some of the methods created by sleep researchers are modified versions of other sleep-training methods. So, for example, Ferber's "ignore but check" method (see Chapter 7 for more information) is a modification of the "ignore it" approach (see Chapter 6 for more information).

In a similar sense, you can combine various techniques from different methods to create your own sleep-training approach. For example, you might combine having a consistent bedtime routine (see Chapters 8 and 11) with a behavior-modification strategy like "ignoring but checking" (see Chapter 7).

You never know—maybe in 20 years people will be talking about "Your Last Name Here"-izing their babies, the way they talk about "Ferber"-izing them now!

What It Is

Let's start with what it isn't, shall we? The combined approach isn't just a mishmash of various techniques and strategies cribbed at random from the different sleep-training methods. ("I'll have the 'ignore but check' method to start, followed by the 'bedtime routines' approach, with a little 'co-sleeping' on the side, and a nice bottle of 'scheduled awakenings.'") Doing that would most likely result in an ineffective approach, not to mention an extremely confused baby.

Instead, there are two basic ways of combining approaches:

◆ You can use one method as a framework with strategies borrowed from other methods to help that basic method work better for you; or,

◆ Because many methods are designed to treat either sleep-onset *or* night-waking problems, if you have a child who has both issues, you may need to use two different techniques to solve both problems.

Infant Almanac

Using the combining approach enables you to continue using a particular sleep-training method instead of abandoning it when you have a setback. You just modify the approach and continue.

How It Works

How do you do it? For example, you could decide to use the "ignore it" method described in Chapter 6, but also apply some of the principles of the "bedtime routine" approach (see Chapter 11). That way, you'd be using the "ignore it" approach as the framework for your sleep-training approach, but you'd be adding to it in order to create a better chance of success for you and your baby.

Why bother? Because combining these two approaches means that even if your baby cries for long periods of time at bedtime, you don't have to give up the "ignore it" method that you've chosen for your child's sleep training.

Instead, you might try changing some aspect of the routine—your bedtime ritual, for example, or the bedtime schedule you set for your child. Doing so may help your child settle down without the need to cry so much.

Unhappy Baby Alert

Going back and forth between methods may result in confusing your baby. Combining strategies isn't about trying one method and then another, but rather combining different strategies from different approaches to make a method that works best for you and your baby.

Combining approaches this way reinforces what you're doing and makes it more likely that you'll stick with the sleep-training method and reach success.

Want more? Suppose your baby has two sleep issues—she has trouble falling asleep at night, and she has more night wakings than you can stand. You want to use Ferber's "ignore but check" method (described in Chapter 7), but after listening to your baby cry at bedtime, you don't have the nerves of steel to also listen to her cry when she wakes at night.

To solve this dilemma, use the "ignore but check" method to help your baby settle at night and then use the "scheduled awakenings" approach (see Chapter 10) to deal with night wakings. You would put your baby to bed and let her cry for gradually longer periods of time, while following the "scheduled awakenings" recommendation to wake your baby up at scheduled intervals throughout the night to gradually reduce the number of night wakings. This would solve your middle-of-the-night nerve problem, and eventually your baby will learn to self-soothe.

And in This Corner: Supporters of This Approach

Using combined strategies is often the way that sleep doctors take care of young children's sleep problems in a sensitive way. Often one method will only solve one problem. Some children have more than one sleep issue.

Dr. Jodi Mindell (see Chapter 8 for more about her) advocates a combined approach of establishing bedtime routines with an "ignore but check" method, for example.

Using This Approach

Consider combining approaches if you have reservations about some aspect of a sleep-training approach that otherwise appeals to you.

You can also consider the combined approach if you're using one of the methods described and it's *almost* working for you, but not quite. A little tweak, some fairy dust from another method, and voilá! You could have a sleep-training method that sends your little one off to dreamland with no problems.

Step-by-Step

Combining approaches doesn't have to be as complicated as it may sound. Follow these play-by-play strategies, and you'll be set.

◆ First, you'll need to educate yourself about the various approaches to understand how they can work together.

◆ Next, you'll want to identify why the approach you're using (or want to use) isn't working the way you want it to. From this analysis you can determine the solution.

◆ Finally, you'll want to assess whether or not your combined-methods approach is working the way you want it to by asking these questions:

Does it solve the problem?

Does it create a new problem?

How do I feel about it?

How does my baby/child seem to feel about it?

If your combined approach solves your original problem without creating a new one, and you and your baby tolerate it reasonably well, then your work here is done.

But if your assessment shows that the approach has created a new problem or that you're uncomfortable with the way things are working out, then you'll want to reconsider your means and methods and try another approach.

Melissa's Mindset

You'll notice that some sleep-training approaches are more compatible with each other than others. "Ignoring it" and "sharing the bed," for example, are going to clash instead of complement each other—not least because they represent very different parenting philosophies. A good rule of thumb to remember is that the approaches described in Part 2 of this book have similar parenting philosophies, while those described in Part 3 share similar philosophies.

Putting the Pieces Together

You've done your research and figured out the basics of each of the sleep-training approaches. Now you have to put them together. Where to start?

Use these sample combined approaches as starting points for your own decision making:

Sample Concern #1: You've heard your friends have had great success with the "scheduled awakenings" approach for their baby's night-waking problem, and you're willing to try it, but you need more guidance in how to get your baby to go to sleep in the first place.

Solution: Choose a complementary approach, such as "ignore but be there" (Chapter 8).

Why it works: In both approaches, the parent is trying to shape the baby's behavior instead of simply reacting to it. Because scheduled awakenings can only be done once the baby is asleep, if your precious one has trouble falling asleep on her own in addition to waking at all hours of the night, you'll need to choose a bedtime strategy as well. In this case, a combined approach would be necessary, rather than simply a preference.

Sample Concern #2: You've been co-sleeping with your baby and you love the feeling of intimacy and closeness you have, but after 18 months, you're still breastfeeding every few hours—and if you don't get 8 full hours soon, you won't be responsible for your behavior.

Solution: In order to break the association your child has developed between nursing and sleeping, you might try changing the bedtime and nighttime waking routine (see Chapter 10) and try to develop positive sleep associations (see Chapter 13).

Why it works: The baby has gotten used to falling asleep at the breast and now needs to nurse every time he wakes up in order to get himself back to sleep. Once the association between nursing and falling asleep has been broken and more positive sleep associations have been made, the child will be better able to soothe himself at night when he wakes up.

Sample Concern #3: You used the "ignore but check" method (see Chapter 7) when your child was younger and it worked fine, but now that she's a toddler and mobile, you have trouble getting her to go to bed in the first place, not to mention getting her to stay there. Trying to ignore it just leads to battles as she climbs out of bed and demands your attention no matter what you do.

Solution: Try combining the Ferber method (ignore but check) with the "bedtime routine" approach (see Chapter 11 for more information).

Why it works: The "bedtime routine" approach can help you deal with toddler resistance to bedtime by showing your toddler that bedtime can be good. Thus, she'll (eventually) go to bed with fewer problems, and fall asleep more quickly. Then you can use Ferber's "ignore but check" method for any night wakings that persist.

Sample Concern #4: You may feel that waiting it out is the best strategy for your young baby. But you're concerned that without any direction at all, the baby might be in grad school before he sleeps through the night.

Solution: Combine the "wait it out" approach (described in Chapter 14) with the bedtime routines that are popular in the "ignore it" approaches (Chapters 6, 7, and 8).

Why it works: Your child gets accustomed to a bedtime routine and is encouraged to learn to sleep by himself, but you don't have to listen to tears or expect your child to perform beyond what you think he's capable of performing.

Challenges You'll Encounter

When you try to combine approaches, one challenge you're likely to run into is that you may not have a clear idea about what needs to be changed with your current approach. In that case, you might end up adding strategies that don't solve the problem.

Be sure you understand what your child's sleep issue is—for example, trouble falling asleep at bedtime—and use an approach that is designed to fix that problem. In other words, the "scheduled awakenings" approach is not going to help you with bedtime resistance.

Another challenge is that combining approaches can add a layer of complexity to an already far-from-simple method.

Advantages to This Approach

The beauty of combining approaches is that you don't have to blindly follow a sleep-training method if you disagree with some aspects of it. You can tailor it to suit your parenting philosophy and personal choices.

In addition, you can combine strategies to provide the best solution for your child's sleep problems, just like sleep specialists do.

Drawbacks to This Approach

Despite your best intentions, you might well end up with a mishmash of techniques and strategies that doesn't really serve any purpose.

Melissa's Mindset

Don't forget that you can consult a sleep specialist for further help instead of trying to solve every problem on your own!

Another potential problem is that you might end up switching from one method to another instead of using them together. Be sure you understand what you're trying to do when combining approaches.

What Parents Say About This Approach

Jill combined the Ferber method with scheduled awakenings when she was blessed with triplets. (We tell her "scheduled awakenings" story in Chapter 10.)

In addition to the scheduled awakenings to help deal with night wakings, Jill first used Ferber's "ignore but check" approach (see Chapter 7) to help with bedtime sleep issues, including adhering to a schedule and crying it out. "I was religious about naps. The better the naps, the better the sleep at night. I also found that the seemingly paradoxical statement, 'sleep begets sleep,' is true. The more they slept during the day, the more they slept at night.

"Sure, there were tough times. [When] we employed the 'cry it out' method, we would carefully monitor how long a baby would cry, and let the kid go no more than 10 minutes. (This was after a few months of age.) I would cry sometimes, too, and think how cruel a mother I was … but then people would say, 'but you *have* to do that—you have triplets!' To which I always responded, 'But *all* mothers have to sleep!'"

The combined approach worked extremely well for Jill and her three babies because she chose compatible approaches and adhered to them faithfully (even when she cried, too!).

The Least You Need to Know

♦ Combining approaches is a reasonable way to deal with shortcomings in a given sleep-training method.

♦ Combining methods enables you to create an approach that will work for you and your baby.

♦ Choosing compatible approaches increases your likelihood of success, as sleep specialists know.

♦ Just as two heads are better than one, two approaches can be better than one!

4

My Baby's Not a Baby! Sleep Training for Children

Let's face it, sometimes we let the baby run the show and we do whatever it takes to let him (and us) get some sleep. But as your child grows older, you may feel the need to deal with sleep disruptions and problems. Or, you may have taught your baby good sleep habits, but now that he's older, he has trouble falling asleep.

In this part, we'll discuss how to adapt sleep-training methods for older children and we'll explain why your child may be having more sleep interruptions and disruptions as he gets older.

Chapter

16

Tucking Toddlers In (Ages 1–3)

In This Chapter

- ◆ Understanding your toddler's new attitude toward sleep
- ◆ Recognizing and dealing with sleep disruptions
- ◆ Encouraging healthy napping
- ◆ Creating a calming bedtime routine

In this chapter, we'll show how to cope with your toddler's new sleep woes. We'll describe why the terrible 2s (and threatening 3s) create sleep challenges for your toddler—and for you.

Never fear: it's not all bad news. We'll also offer some suggestions for dealing with those sleep challenges.

We'll show you how to choose an effective sleep-training method for your toddler and how to modify the most popular approaches to work with your young'un.

Why Toddlers Have Sleep Troubles

As your baby morphs into a toddler, you'll start dealing with new kinds of problems. Toddlers test you and push your limits (they also push your buttons). So you can expect to start having some battles over sleep.

Melissa's Mindset

Toddlers test their parents because they are trying to become more independent and want to know where their boundaries are. Believe it or not, the trials they put you through are developmentally appropriate and a sign that you should be proud! Your completely dependent infant is growing up right on track. The best medicine for a testy toddler is consistency. By being consistent in as many realms as possible—including sleep—parents teach their toddlers where the boundaries are and what's not worth testing.

At bedtime, they'll need to go to the potty "one more time" 10 times (if you let them). Setting limits can help curb potential bedtime brouhahas before they happen, but standing strong at bedtime won't make that much of a difference if you cave at other times of day. Now more than ever you need to be consistent in your schedule, expectations, and discipline.

Infant Almanac

Toddlers often need extra help with transitions. Be sure to remind them what the bedtime rules are (and yes, you have to remind them every single night, and more than once): "You can have one trip to the potty and one glass of water."

In addition, toddlers start to be aware of the nightmares they experience. (Infants probably have nightmares as well but they're unable to tell us about them.) Because of your toddler's growing maturity, she identifies those bad dreams as frightening and remembers them, but doesn't understand that those alternate realities are not real. Remember: to her they *are* real.

As a result, your toddler may be afraid of going to sleep (because she's afraid of having nightmares), or she may wake up from a nightmare and have difficulty going back to sleep without help and reassurance from you.

Because their brains and bodies are changing, the sleep patterns toddlers had as babies will change. As they reach various developmental milestones, it may seem as if they "unlearn" some of their formerly mastered behavior. A 2-year-old who was sleeping through the night starts verbalizing more and more—and suddenly quits sleeping through the night. Although normal, it can be disconcerting to parents who thought night patrol was pretty much done.

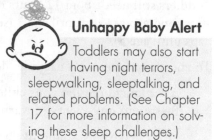

Unhappy Baby Alert

Toddlers may also start having night terrors, sleepwalking, sleeptalking, and related problems. (See Chapter 17 for more information on solving these sleep challenges.)

Underlying Medical Conditions

Toddlers may also have medical problems that contribute to sleep difficulties:

- Central sleep apnea (breathing cessation), while rare, can occur in toddlers and disrupt sleep.

- Enlarged tonsils and adenoids may block breathing, leading to obstructive sleep apnea.

- Allergies may cause swelling of nasal tissues and cause breathing difficulties.

- Obesity can cause obstructive sleep apnea.

Infant Almanac

For children, the most common treatment for obstructive sleep apnea is having tonsils and adenoids removed.

Infant Almanac

Snoring is a sign of potential breathing problems. The occasional snore is nothing to worry about, but heavy snoring, prolonged snoring, and persistent snoring may indicate that a trip to the pediatrician is in order.

Consulting a pediatrician and/or a sleep specialist will help you handle sleep problems that have a medical origin.

Napping Do's and Don'ts

Toddlers will often have nighttime sleep problems if they're not getting enough sleep during the day. So bedtime difficulties may have their origin in poor napping.

Toddlers still need about 12 hours of sleep every day. And they need an afternoon nap at least until age 3 (some kids continue to need afternoon naps until age 5).

To encourage afternoon napping, do the following:

- After lunch, remind your child that nap time is around the corner. Be sure to give plenty of warning.

- Don't make naps sound like a punishment and never use the bed, or bedroom, or going to sleep, as a punishment.

- Remove your child from the action.

- Use naptime rituals to encourage sleep. Doing things like saying "night, night" to the dog, cat, fish, or the photographs on the wall can be part of this kind of routine, as could reading a story, listening to soft music and the like.

Unhappy Baby Alert

A toddler who continues to have two naps a day may have trouble sleeping at night. Most toddlers have consolidated daytime sleep into one afternoon nap by the age of 2. A single nap that ends by mid-afternoon won't make it harder for your toddler to sleep at night. It may actually *improve* his nighttime sleep.

Eliminating the morning nap can help your child sleep better during his afternoon nap and at night. To wean your child to one nap, try the following:

1. Move the morning nap to later in the day.

2. Move the afternoon nap earlier.

3. Move naps in 15-minute increments every few days.

4. Eventually the two naps will merge into one.

Waking with the Roosters

Early-morning waking is a common sleep problem among toddlers. To help prevent it (and deal with it), do the following:

- Encourage the toddler to safely play alone in her room instead of coming to get you or you going to get her right away. You may need to help her by giving her a signal: "When the sun comes up, you may get out of bed and come to get me."

♦ Make sure your toddler is getting sufficient rest—not enough sleep causes sleep problems.

♦ Try shortening or eliminating a nap if the child is getting sufficient sleep and is ready to wake up at dawn.

♦ End the afternoon nap by 3 P.M.

♦ Try a slightly later bedtime.

♦ Keep the room dark and quiet—heavy shades can prevent morning sunlight from waking the child.

Melissa's Mindset

A child who knows her numbers may benefit from a digital clock in her room to help in knowing when it's "ok" to get out of bed and come into her parents' room. "When the clock says 6-3-0 then it's ok to come out of your room." My brother used this technique in Arizona (and set the clock to Eastern Standard time).

Banging Your Head

Or rather, your toddler is banging his. You put your kid to bed and pretty soon your hear "thump ... thump ... thump" as your little one bumps his head against the wall. Or you wake up to the lullaby of "smack ... smack ... smack" as your child tries to lull himself back to sleep by headbutting the crib headboard at 3 A.M.

If your child is otherwise healthy and developing appropriately, headbanging is normal. Remember ...

Infant Almanac

Headbanging sometimes occurs in children ages 1 to 3 because it soothes the child (although it's alarming to parents).

♦ It may only last a few weeks until your toddler develops a better way of soothing herself back to sleep.

♦ It usually goes away on its own.

♦ Like many things your toddler does, the more you struggle with it, the more likely you'll reinforce the behavior instead of eliminating it.

♦ Offer alternatives: a lovey, a rock in the rocking chair—but don't make a big production of it.

However, there are circumstances when you should seek help for head-banging, such as when it …

♦ Lasts for more than 15 minutes.

♦ Is repeated throughout the night and during the day while the child is awake.

> **Unhappy Baby Alert**
>
> If your child is over age 3 and still engaging in headbanging, it is less likely to go away on its own. Consult a pediatrician for further advice.

♦ Does not go away after 18 months.

♦ Causes injury.

♦ Occurs in a child with medical problems, who is not developing appropriately, or who is under stress.

Got Teeth?

Some children grind or gnash their teeth at night—as many as 50 percent of children have this problem. Usually it's mild and may not require any intervention. If it's frequent and violent, though, it can cause jaw problems, headaches, damaged teeth, earaches, facial pain, tooth sensitivity, and other problems.

> **Infant Almanac**
>
> If your toddler grinds his teeth, you may be able to hear it when he sleeps.

>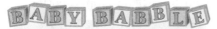
>
> **Bruxism** is the medical term for grinding your teeth.

In young children, *bruxism*, or teeth grinding, may occur because their upper teeth don't fit together well. It can also be related to stress, allergies, and teething. Caffeine may even contribute to the problem.

Most children outgrow teeth grinding before their adult teeth come in. However, be sure to consult your pediatrician if you're concerned about the problem or if it seems to be causing your child pain.

Creating a Bedtime Routine

Toddlers respond well to structure, schedules, and rituals. Because of this, creating a bedtime ritual that you do the same way every single night can help your toddler prepare to fall asleep.

Toddlers find this ritual soothing and reassuring, and it helps them feel some control over the process. It also helps them transition from one activity (play/wakefulness) to another (bed/sleeptime). By reciting the steps of the ritual before you do them ("We need to take a bath, brush your teeth, change into your pajamas, tuck you in bed, read a story, and sing a song"), and then as you do them, you'll encourage your toddler in the transition to bedtime.

You may want to prepare for your toddler's bedtime as early as right after supper. As a general rule of thumb, it's best to avoid rough play, television, and video and computer games after supper.

 Unhappy Baby Alert

Toddlers love ritual so much that they will immediately know if you miss a step and they will be extremely upset. They will also try to add steps to a ritual in order to prolong it. So focus on keeping the bedtime ritual reasonably short—and don't dare to forget a step!

Melissa's Mindset

Although many toddlers now have a TV in their rooms, it is recommended that TV not be used as part of the bedtime ritual. Watching TV is associated with irregular sleep schedules. Having a TV in a child's room creates a habit that may be hard to break and is not good for her sleep.

Transitioning from the Family Bed

If you've been co-sleeping with your baby, you may feel that now that she's a toddler, it's time for her to move to her own bed. Some children will make the transition without parental intervention, but others won't. To encourage the transition, try the following:

♦ Don't use an "ignore it" method for a child who has spent his infancy in a family bed.

- Toddlers love to feel "big," so encourage the child to see sleeping in his own bed as an indication that he's a big boy (having a cool bed to transition to can also help).

- Take it step-by-step and don't think of occasional returns to your bed as disasters.

- Offer a lovey or transitional object.

- Allow the child to sleep in a bed next to yours.

- Put her down in her bed for naps.

- Don't immediately move her to her room at night—give it some time.

- Go to her when she wakes in her room at night (instead of expecting her to come to you).

- After a period of time you can offer verbal reassurance from your room without getting up to go comfort her.

Transitioning from Crib to Bed

When your child becomes a toddler, you naturally begin thinking about moving him from crib to bed. Whether your child is ready depends on his age, size, and maturity level.

Your child might be eager to move to a bed—and you might be eager to see him do so since it's a milestone. But remember that once the child is in a bed of his own he can get out at will, and that makes getting him to sleep (and getting him to go back to sleep after a night waking) more difficult. It is also a safety issue: a toddler roaming the house at night can get into all sorts of trouble. So, be careful what you wish for!

Unhappy Baby Alert

If your toddler is climbing out of her crib, you should move her to a bed or use a crib tent, which will reduce the risk of falls, strangulation, and other hazards.

Follow these rules of thumb for deciding when it's time for your toddler to move to a bed:

- Keep your child in her crib as long as possible. Three years old may be an ideal age to transition.

◆ Check the weight limit on your crib. When your child reaches that weight, you will need to move her to a bed.

◆ Don't move your child to a bed just because a new baby is coming and you want to use the crib. This may make the toddler jealous and resentful of the new baby.

◆ If your child is excited about moving to a bed, follow his lead.

> **Unhappy Baby Alert**
>
> Placing a safety gate across the doorway to the toddler's room prevents him from getting out of bed and wandering around the house, but it also doesn't make him feel abandoned. You might also keep a monitor in the child's room so that you can hear when he is awake.

Choosing the Most Effective Method for Your Toddler

Maybe you used a sleep-training method for your infant but it doesn't work on your toddler. Or your baby was a pretty good sleeper so you never had to worry about sleep training—until your toddler stopped sleeping through the night.

What should you do? How do you choose which approach to use with your toddler?

First, don't fret. While it may be ideal to start sleep-training methods with an older infant, you can use most sleep-training approaches perfectly well with a toddler. The only difference is that a toddler can get out of bed and walk around, and toddlers can be stubborn enough to make extinction methods ("ignore it" and the like, Chapters 6, 7 and 8) harrowing to attempt.

Your first step should be to think about what worked for your toddler when she was a baby. If that approach no longer fills the bill, maybe you don't need to abandon it. Maybe you just need to modify it. (See Chapters 11 and 15 for more on modifying and combining sleep-training approaches.)

If you didn't really use a method, or if you need to find an entirely new approach, consider your toddler's personality and temperament as well as your parenting philosophy. If you've used the family bed and have transitioned your toddler to her own bed, suddenly using the "ignore it" approach is probably going to be too hard on everyone. Instead, choose a "no tears" method such as co-sleeping, changing the routine, or the persistent gentle removal approach, which is more likely to succeed with your child—and with you.

Once your toddler is in her own bed, trying to keep her there at bedtime can be difficult. This is especially true when she is not used to falling asleep on her own.

Dr. Jodi Mindell, a sleep researcher, recommends using a modified "ignore it" method for toddlers. If the toddler is having trouble staying in bed, the parent might conduct the bedtime ritual as usual, and then run "errands" for gradually increasing times, giving praise to the child every time he stays in bed while she is away.

Here is how it works: Dad puts Johnny to bed, and then says he needs to put a load of laundry in the washing machine (a dream husband!) and he'll be right back. Dad returns in 2 minutes (or 30 seconds, depending on the child), sits with Johnny for a few minutes, and then makes up another errand. This time he's gone for longer—perhaps 5 minutes. This strategy continues until Johnny has fallen asleep.

Parents need to remember to always return to the child's room after every errand. There's nothing worse to a child than being told that a parent will return in a given amount of time and not having that happen. Parents might run several errands in one night or just one; the idea is to gradually increase the length of the errands across time so the child learns to stay in bed.

Modifying the Approach

Most of the sleep-training approaches we describe in this book can be used to help toddlers learn to go to sleep and to fall back to sleep after night wakings. However, in some cases you'll need to modify the approach.

Modifying "Ignore It" Methods

"Ignore it" methods are more difficult because you can't just ignore the crying infant by turning up the volume on the television. Your toddler can and will get out of bed and in your face. Because he can climb out of bed and toddle into the living room, you have to make a few modifications. Ferber suggests sitting outside the bedroom door and putting the child back to bed. (See Chapter 7 for more information on this method.) You may also put a gate up (But then be prepared to see your child sleeping on the floor by the gate when you come to get him in the morning.)

A modification of the "ignore but be there" method (see Chapter 8) has you sitting in a chair in the toddler's room, and then moving the chair farther away from the toddler's bed on progressive nights until you're finally out the door.

Modifying "No Tears" Methods

The "no tears" methods don't require a lot of changes because you're reacting to the child's needs (more or less), and it doesn't matter if those needs are presented by a baby crying in a crib or a toddler yanking at your robe.

However, because of the nature of toddlers (limit-pushing little creatures that they are), you may find that you have to be firmer and less flexible in your approach in order to get them to comply.

The Least You Need to Know

- ◆ Toddlers have different sleep challenges from infants.
- ◆ Encouraging the right kind of naps helps toddlers sleep better at night.
- ◆ Creating a bedtime routine makes bedtimes easier for everyone.
- ◆ Sleep-training approaches that work for infants will work for toddlers, too.

Chapter 17

Getting Preschoolers and Schoolagers to Sleep (Ages 3–8)

In This Chapter

- Understanding your young child's sleep challenges
- Recognizing and dealing with sleep disruptions that occur in young children
- Encouraging healthy sleep habits
- Getting the lowdown on nightmares, night terrors, bedwetting, sleepwalking, and other nighttime nuisances

Just when you thought it was safe to assume your sleepytime troubles were over … your young child suddenly develops a firm conviction that monsters, invisible during daylight hours and to adult eyes, creep out from under the bed just as soon as you say goodnight and shut out the lights. Needless to say, your young child does not want to share her room with monsters—and now you have a new problem on your hands.

In this chapter, we'll show you how to tame the boogey monsters so that your little one can get some shut-eye.

We'll also explain how the sleep challenges that young children face are different from those that babies and toddlers encounter—and we'll clue you in on why. We'll let you know what to expect about bedtime battles as your toddler turns into a preschooler and then a schoolager.

And, finally, don't worry—we'll give you some suggestions for combating everything from bedwetting to bedtime resistance, and we'll alert you to those times when you'll need to think about getting Dr. Welby on the case.

Why Young Children Have Sleep Troubles

As toddlers mature into preschoolers and schoolagers, their understanding of how the world works becomes more sophisticated, they become more aware of external events (everything from bullies at school to natural disasters), and they become more aware of their vulnerability.

> **Infant Almanac**
>
> Children's fears transform from imaginary to realistic as they get older, which is why you'll need monster spray one year and child-level discussions of what to do in case of a hurricane the next. "Monster spray" is useful to eradicate the monster problem in many children's rooms, as long as the child does the spraying and believes it will work.

They're also learning to deal with their own aggression, which their teachers and parents now require them to keep under control. So it's common for children to have nighttime fears of the dark, monsters and witches and related riff-raff, peaking at ages 4 to 5. Older children may be afraid of illness, injury, and natural disasters.

Because of these psychological, emotional, and even physical changes, children in this age group may resist going to bed and use lots of delaying and stalling tactics, and may want you to stay with them.

Sometimes these bedtime fears can be addressed by ...

- ◆ Showing your child that the room has no monsters in it—looking in the closet and under the bed.

- ◆ Discussing your child's fear (but not right at bedtime).

Melissa's Mindset

A series of children's books written by Mercer Mayer address children's nighttime fears directly and effectively (*There's a Nightmare in My Closet, There's an Alligator Under My Bed, There's Something in My Attic*). Young children love these stories, and they each vividly deal with a child confronting his or her fears. I like them because they acknowledge the reality of children's fears without dismissing or ridiculing them, are humorous, and assure children that they can effectively conquer their own fears.

♦ Encouraging the use of a security object or lovey—a toy or blanket that comforts the child.

♦ Keeping the household calm, especially at bedtime.

♦ Not dismissing or ridiculing the child's fears.

♦ Not reinforcing the child's fears but noticing when he is being "brave."

♦ Demonstrating positive coping skills.

♦ Encouraging your child to stay in bed despite fears.

♦ Showing relaxation or self-soothing techniques (see Chapter 20 for more information).

Infant Almanac

A child's persistent or unreasonable fears could signal a phobia or anxiety disorder. Consult your pediatrician if you have concerns about fears that seem to be debilitating or if your child seems to be extremely anxious.

Infant Almanac

Children also sometimes associate sleep with death. This association is reinforced when adults use euphemisms like, "We had to put the dog to sleep." If someone close to the child has died recently, use kid-level language to explain: "Grandpa was very sick. He had a heart attack and died." Even if you're trying to make the event less traumatic, try to avoid making statements like, "He died peacefully in his sleep"—even if he did.

Notes on Napping

Some children need an afternoon nap up to age 5, especially when newly involved in activities that are mentally or physically tiring, like beginning preschool.

But if your child continues napping after age 5, it may signal that she is not getting adequate sleep at night or is suffering from an underlying medical condition that needs treatment.

Encourage an earlier bedtime for the sleep-deprived child, and consider these possible causes:

◆ Obstructive sleep apnea may cause daytime drowsiness.

◆ Medications can cause daytime sleepiness.

◆ Depression and other psychological disorders may cause sleepiness.

◆ Narcolepsy and other neurological disorders may cause daytime drowsiness.

◆ Certain physical disorders can cause fatigue during the day.

You may want to consult your pediatrician or a sleep clinician if your child has more than occasional daytime sleepiness.

Nightmares and Dreams

Nightmares are scary dreams that occur during *REM sleep* They may wake your child and cause him to cry. Children ages 4 to 6 tend to have more nightmares because of their growing independence and emotional development, and also because of their increased use of imagination. During the day they may play Superman, but they can feel small and defenseless at night.

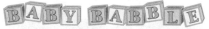

REM sleep is the sleep stage in which most dreams occur. Although periods of REM sleep occur throughout the night, it is concentrated in the early-morning hours. See Chapter 2 for more information on REM and non-REM sleep.

Young children don't really understand that dreams aren't real, so even a vivid dream that's not a nightmare can be upsetting. By the age of 6 or 7 most children are less upset by their dreams and nightmares, although occasionally they will still be frightened by one.

If your child is under a lot of stress, she may have more nightmares. Scary things that have happened during the day can become fodder for nightmares. For example, if a dog chased her after school, she may have a nightmare about the experience.

Infant Almanac

Nightmares may make a child not want to go to bed, so they can cause sleep disruption. Take steps to help reassure your child if she is prone to nightmares.

Here are some strategies for dealing with nightmares:

♦ Offer comfort and reassurance after a nightmare.

♦ Discuss any daytime scares (e.g., the dog chasing her after school) and offer reassurance—but not just before bed.

♦ Place a nightlight in the bedroom (preferably not one that casts creepy shadows on the wall).

♦ Remind your child how to self-soothe (for example, think comforting thoughts or say a prayer—see Chapter 20).

♦ Reduce pressures on your child and teach positive stress-coping skills.

♦ Supervise television, movies, and videogames, and rule out those that are too exciting, scary, or violent.

Night Terrors

Night terrors are different from nightmares. They occur during *deep sleep* and the child does not remember them. They're alarming to parents because the child may scream, cry, and/or thrash around on the bed but does not respond to you when you go to him.

Infant Almanac

Here's a rule of thumb to remember: if the child is more upset, then it's a nightmare; if you're more upset, then it's a night terror.

Night terrors are most common in children aged 3–6, and may be associated with stress in the child's life. Causes include sleep deprivation, illnesses, changes in routine, or a new environment. They generally decrease in frequency as the child gets older, and go away on their own.

Here are things to remember:

◆ Don't try to awaken the child—he is still basically asleep during the episode and will lie down and calm down by himself eventually; waking him can cause him to be extremely confused and disoriented. More important, trying to wake the child can prolong the event.

◆ Night terrors are not seizures.

◆ They are not dangerous unless your child thrashes about in a way that could hurt her.

◆ Don't restrain your child, but keep the area around him clear.

◆ Consult a pediatrician or sleep specialist if you're concerned or if the night terrors are frequent and persistent.

BABY BABBLE

A **night terror,** or "sleep terror," because they don't only happen during the night, is a sleep disorder (known in the sleep world as a type of "parasomnia") that happens in deep sleep and is characterized by the child sitting upright and screaming, about 90 minutes to 2 hours after falling asleep. The child appears to be frightened and is impossible to console.

Deep sleep refers to stages 3 and 4 of nonrapid eye movement (NREM or non-REM) sleep. Although this type of sleep recurs throughout the night, it's concentrated toward the beginning of nighttime sleep. That's why most night terrors occur in the first couple of hours after the child falls asleep. See Chapter 2 for more information on REM and non-REM sleep.

Bedwetting

Bedwetting is common up to about age 5 and occurs occasionally even in older children. Doctors don't consider it a problem unless it continues once the child has reached 5 years old or begins after the child has been able to remain dry at night for some time. In the meantime, diapers and pullups can be used at night, as can plastic or vinyl mattress protectors.

It's thought that children wet at night either because they're unable to let their bladder become full before needing to void or they aren't able to rouse themselves when their bladder is full.

Parents may be able to help their bedwetting child by following these steps:

◆ Encourage the child to get more sleep. More sleep means the child sleeps less deeply and can wake completely to use the bathroom instead of wetting in bed.

Melissa's Mindset

Bedwetting, or "sleep enuresis," occurs in about 30 percent of 4-year-olds, 10 percent of 5-year-olds, 5 percent of 10-year-olds, and 3 percent of 12-year-olds. It is more common in boys and is thought to be at least partly genetic. So if a parent was a bed-wetter, the child is more likely to be one as well. Bedwetting happens mostly in deep sleep.

◆ Reduce the amount of liquids given after supper.

◆ Encourage a few low-pressure trips to the potty before bed.

◆ Place a potty chair in the child's room—and have the child participate in choosing it.

◆ Wake the child to use the potty just before you go to bed.

Because bedwetting usually goes away as your child gets older, check with your pediatrician about your child's bedwetting if …

◆ Your child is 5 or older.

Infant Almanac

The most important thing to remember about bedwetting is this: don't make an issue of it by punishing or shaming the child. It's not something your child can control.

◆ Your child was dry for at least 6 months before bedwetting started, as this is likely caused by a medical problem such as a urinary tract infection.

◆ You feel concerned about how to handle the problem, are worried about possible underlying conditions, or feel frustrated with the problem.

To help solve the problem, your pediatrician may recommend one of the following strategies:

◆ An alerting device—a sensor detects moisture on the sheets and sets off an alarm to wake the child. It may help the child learn to wake before wetting.

◆ Dry training—requires waking the child repeatedly at night to use the toilet. It's disruptive to the child (not to mention you) but can be successful. It's important that the child not feel punished if using this technique.

◆ Bladder training—teaching the child to hold larger amounts of water during the daytime and to exert better control over starting and stopping urination.

◆ Medication—an anti-diuretic may help the child stay dry for short periods of time but does not solve the bed-wetting problem. May be good for a sleepover or vacation but is not a cure.

Sleepwalking and Sleeptalking

Melissa's Mindset

Sleepwalking is known in the sleep world as "somnambulism" and is experienced by as many as 15 percent of children at least once. It's most common in children ages 4–8 and often goes away on its own.

Sleepwalking and sleeptalking, like night terrors, occur during deep sleep. Sleeptalking is more common than sleepwalking and has a similar cause, but of course it's not as alarming to parents as sleepwalking is.

If you have a child who sleepwalks, you'll want to take some safety precautions:

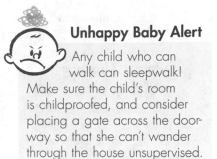

Unhappy Baby Alert

Any child who can walk can sleepwalk! Make sure the child's room is childproofed, and consider placing a gate across the doorway so that she can't wander through the house unsupervised.

◆ Place a nightlight in her room and in nearby hallways.

◆ Consider putting an alarm on the bedroom door to alert you to her nighttime wanderings.

◆ Keep floors clear.

◆ Keep windows and doors shut and locked.

◆ Place a gate across stairways.

◆ Don't restrain, slap, shake, or shout at a sleepwalking child; gently guide him back to bed.

◆ Don't embarrass, frighten, or pressure a child who sleepwalks. Just state the safety precautions you're taking so that he understands why you're doing what you're doing.

Infant Almanac

Sleepwalking in children over age 6 may be caused by stress, fever, or sleep deprivation. Encouraging good sleep habits and helping the child learn positive stress-coping techniques can reduce or eliminate the problem.

◆ Don't talk to the child about his sleep walking the next day. Children may become frightened that it will happen again and not want to go to sleep. This will only make the problem worse, because sleep walking occurs more often when children are sleep deprived.

Underlying Medical Conditions

Young children may also have medical problems that contribute to sleep difficulties. One of the most common medical sleep problems for children is obstructive sleep apnea syndrome (OSAS). It is estimated that between 5 to 6 percent of children have OSAS. As discussed in Chapter 2, enlarged tonsils and adenoids can cause OSAS, as can obesity. If your child snores regularly and loudly, it is essential to discuss this with your pediatrician, as this may be a sign that your child has OSAS. OSAS can cause daytime sleepiness as well as ADHD-like symptoms that will go away with treatment.

> **Infant Almanac**
>
> Medical problems that interfere with breathing and disrupt sleep are often signaled by snoring. If your child snores persistently, it may be a sign of an underlying medical problem that should be treated.

Other medical conditions such as allergies or respiratory infections can cause breathing difficulties during sleep as well. If you suspect your child has any of these conditions, consult your pediatrician.

Creating a Bedtime Routine

Poor sleep is one of the most common problems children at this age have, and the reason why children have poor sleep is because of their poor sleep habits. But habits can be changed! Poor sleep habits can often be overcome by taking these steps:

- ◆ Keep a set schedule for your young child.

- ◆ Maintain regular wake- and bedtimes.

- ◆ Don't change wake- and bedtimes over the weekend.

- ◆ Don't overschedule your child.

- ◆ Reduce television, computer, and videogame time, especially before bed.

- ◆ Make your child's bedroom comfortable and appealing for sleep.

- ◆ Make sleep a priority for yourself as well as for your child.

> **Infant Almanac**
>
> Eliminating caffeine from your child's diet can help prevent sleep problems. Caffeine is a stimulant that may disrupt your child's sleep-wake cycle.

Keeping a consistent bedtime routine helps. Your preschooler and schoolager will do better with a specific routine that signals the transition from wake to sleep. At this age, they can help you decide what the routine consists of, and may be able to do most of it themselves without too much help from you.

It's usually a good idea to wind down the day after supper so that not a lot of action is going on just before bedtime. Help your child with his homework (if applicable), play some calm music, put toys away, get the house ready for bed (close curtains, clear clutter, shut off unnecessary lights). Then a warm bath, a sip of milk, a quiet story, and whatever else your child needs to make the transition—and it's off to bed.

The Three Rs: Resisting, Refusing, and Requests

When children hit the preschool years, they become masters of putting off bedtime as long as possible They resist bedtime, refuse to go to bed, and make incessant requests for more water, more stories, more potty time. Here are some of the causes of the three Rs:

- Lack of limits/discipline in this and other areas
- Conflicting parenting styles—children sense that parents aren't in agreement and push boundaries
- Age—younger children have more difficulty complying
- Room-sharing
- Stress, including family tension and anxiety
- Lack of routine schedule
- Side effect of medications

But you're not at the mercy of the three Rs. You can take a few steps to solve the problem:

- Check in with your child.
- Stay calm despite getting your buttons pushed
- Don't lock your child in the room—this creates a bigger problem and more struggles.
- Reward your child for staying in her bed.
- Be consistent and firm about bedtime—make sure the family understands the rules and the adults enforce them.
- Set limits at bedtime and other times.

If your child needs your attention to fall asleep and this is a problem for you, you may need to change her sleep associations so that she doesn't associate you with falling asleep. See Chapter 20 for more information on how she can learn to soothe herself to sleep.

Wake Up, Sleepyhead

Parents of preschoolers who bound out of bed at 5 a.m. every morning may not believe it, but some children have difficulty waking up at a regular time every morning—like in time to get ready for school.

If your child is having difficulty waking at a regular time, try these strategies:

- Set an earlier bedtime. Don't introduce it suddenly; move the child's bedtime back in 5- or 10-minute increments until you find the best bedtime.

- Let the sun shine in—open curtains and blinds at waketime to stimulate your child.

- Set the alarm for the child's actual wake-up time—no snooze alarm allowed. When the alarm goes off, it's time to get out of bed.

Trouble Falling Asleep

Not surprising, the same children who have trouble waking up in the morning often have trouble falling asleep at night. Because they have trouble falling asleep, they don't get enough rest, and thus the struggle to get them dressed and to get some breakfast into them before they head off for school.

For children who have difficulty falling asleep, try the following strategies:

- Avoid naps. Encourage your child to stay awake until bedtime.

- Create a routine: wake up and go to bed at set times every day, including weekends.

- Use the bed for sleep only, not for reading or playing video games or watching TV.

♦ Exercise daily (but not too close to bedtime).

♦ A small snack before bed can help encourage sleepiness.

In addition, your child might benefit from the "positive bedtime routines" approach as described in Chapter 11, which requires a later bedtime so that the child starts falling asleep shortly after going to bed.

Choosing the Most Effective Method for Your Preschooler and Schoolager

Remember that the biggest problems with this age group have to do with going to sleep rather than with night waking. So, effective methods include those that address the going-to-bed issue, such as the "extinction" methods (Chapters 6–8).

The most important thing to remember is to establish or maintain healthy *sleep hygiene* for your preschool and young school-age child. That means helping your child to keep a regular bedtime, a relaxing bedtime routine, and a good sleep environment (free from distractions such as TV or computer).

> **BABY BABBLE**
>
> **Sleep hygiene** means good sleep habits that ensure that your child eventually learns to fall asleep on his own in a reasonable amount of time and can soothe himself back to sleep after night wakings.

As with toddlers, if your preschooler has not yet learned to put herself to sleep at night on her own, you may need to use a sleep-training approach that focuses on teaching her to fall asleep on her own. See Chapter 16 for information on modifying "ignore it" methods to work for older children.

> **Infant Almanac**
>
> Preschoolers and school-agers still need between 10 and 12 hours of sleep a day, so good sleep habits are essential. Maintaining—or establishing—good sleep habits now will help you and your child during the next round of development ... but more on that in Chapter 18.

Modifying the Approach

Because children of this age are dealing more with nightmares and fears about going to bed, it may be necessary for parents to add some techniques to their sleep-training approach in order to help children deal with these fears.

For example, in establishing a bedtime routine, parents might add a step such as "check under bed and in closet for monsters" to the routine (in between "brush teeth" and "read a bedtime story").

The Least You Need to Know

- ◆ Preschool and school-age children have some different sleep challenges from babies and toddlers.

- ◆ Young children are prone to nightmares, night terrors, and sleep-walking—all of which can be alarming to parents and can be disruptive to children, especially if they cause disruption or deprivation of sleep.

- ◆ Creating routines and setting limits will help reduce bedtime battles.

- ◆ Night fears are common among children this age and can make them resist bedtime.

Chapter 18

Convincing the Older Child to Get Some Zzzzs (Ages 8–12)

In This Chapter

- Understanding your older child's sleep challenges
- Recognizing and dealing with sleep disruptions that affect older children
- Developing good sleep habits
- Creating a plan for your older child

When your pediatrician said you might have trouble getting your baby to sleep through the night, you probably didn't think he meant your 10-year-old "baby." But older children have sleep problems, too—in fact, older children are the sleepiest children of all, according to many studies.

Some of their sleep problems are the result of bad habits that started when they were younger. Other difficulties are unique to older children. In any case, many sleep problems can be solved with some patience and a little knowledge.

In this chapter, we'll give you that knowledge (though we can't help you out with the patience). We'll describe sleep problems that older children have and how they can be treated, and we'll give you suggestions for helping your older child develop good sleep habits that will help her the rest of her life. And for those problems that you can't fix on your own, we'll let you know when to seek the help of a sleep specialist.

> **Infant Almanac**
>
> The older child still needs 10–11 hours of sleep at night, but most don't get enough. Studies show that older children get much less sleep than they really need to function well during the day.

When Your Older Child Doesn't Get Enough Sleep

In their eagerness to cram as much as they can into any given day, older children often neglect their sleep. While this may not seem like a big problem—you're likely running on less sleep than you need, too—sleep deprivation is a very big problem.

Making Sleep a Priority

Sleep should be a priority for older children, just as it is for younger children. Not enough sleep causes many difficulties, such as the following:

- Difficulty controlling emotions
- Changes in mood
- Lack of focus
- Impaired academic ability
- Greater tendency to engage in high-risk behavior
- Decrease in motor skill
- Decrease in concentration and reaction time
- Weight gain

◆ Poor judgment

◆ Loss of motivation

◆ Possible increased risk of suicide

Unhappy Baby Alert

Sleep-deprived children can fall asleep for a few seconds at a time without even realizing they've done so!

Sleep Deprived or Doing Fine?

How can you tell if your child is sleep deprived? It can be difficult to tell if your older child is getting enough sleep. In general, your child is getting enough sleep if ...

◆ He falls asleep within 15 minutes of going to bed—as in younger children, overtired older children have trouble falling asleep.

◆ She wakes up easily in the morning and does not need to be nagged several times to get out of bed.

Infant Almanac

A smart way to check on potential sleep deprivation in your older child is to ask your child's teacher if your child is showing signs of sleepiness at school.

◆ He is awake and alert all day and does not need a nap, not even during World History class.

Melissa's Mindset

One of the most interesting findings from sleep research in recent years has been the discovery that some cases of diagnosed Attention Deficit-Hyperactivity Disorder (ADHD) are actually a result of insufficient or poor-quality sleep. Curing the sleep problem makes the symptoms of ADHD disappear. If your child has been diagnosed with ADHD and has not been evaluated for a sleep problem, you might consider finding a sleep specialist to evaluate your child.

A sleep-deprived child is likely to experience some of the following symptoms:

◆ Yawning throughout the day

◆ Lack of energy

◆ Lack of interest in formerly enjoyed activities

- Grogginess during the day
- Temper tantrums
- Blurred vision
- Appetite changes
- Clumsiness

Infant Almanac

Some of the symptoms of sleep deprivation are similar to those for depression and other medical problems. Have your child evaluated by a sleep specialist, a physician, or a psychologist instead of assuming that the problem will solve itself.

- Hyperactivity or inattentiveness
- Aggression
- Mood swings

If you notice these symptoms in your child, your first step should be to encourage more sleep and better sleep habits. An excellent way to do this is to model good sleep habits yourself!

Why Older Children Have Sleep Troubles

Just as preschoolers and young schoolagers have more sleep difficulties as their understanding of the way the world works becomes more sophisticated, older children may also have sleep difficulties related to their connection to the world around them.

As they mature, older children become more aware of violence, disasters, and threats to themselves (and their loved ones). They realize that they can't control everything and this can cause stress and fear.

Older children are more likely to have "realistic" fears that make it hard for them to sleep. Such fears are common in children this age and peak between the ages of 9 and 11. These fears are real, though unlikely to happen. For example, your child may have trouble falling asleep because she's afraid of a hurricane. Unlike a monster under the bed, you can't tell your 11-year-old that there's no such thing as natural disasters.

Reassuring your frightened older child can help, but she will probably be even more comforted by concrete plans. So, for example, you can go over the family safety plan for fires or tornadoes (or whatever is pertinent to your particular situation). Some experts recommend a self-defense course for children worried about personal safety. These steps can help your child sleep easier at night.

BABY BABBLE

Nighttime panic, which is more intense than the nighttime fears many older children experience, is more complicated and may require counseling to address.

Melissa's Mindset

Children who watch a lot of TV often perceive the world as a more dangerous place than it really is. Sometimes, limiting TV time can help to eliminate or reduce the amount of fear your child experiences. This is not to say that you need to or should shield your child from all bad experiences in the world, but limiting his exposure to TV (which tends to focus on the negative) will help, as will discussing fears factually and logically.

Older Children and Sleep Disruptions

As children enter early adolescence, their body rhythms change, making them want to go to bed later. Although some reasons for wanting to stay up later are not biological, there is clear evidence that older children's body clocks change. At least part of the older child's desire to stay up later is natural. In the sleep world, this is known as "delayed sleep phase."

Often, as children's bodies are telling them to stay up later and wake up later, school start times are getting earlier and earlier. This can cause sleep deprivation and the harmful symptoms we described earlier.

Older children may have other sleep disruptions that prevent a solid night's sleep. Here are some common ones:

Infant Almanac

In some communities, school start times have been adjusted later to recognize the biological shift that older children go through. Often, this results in happier children, fewer discipline problems, and better grades.

- ◆ Insomnia, or trouble falling asleep no matter what time the child goes to bed. Children with insomnia don't have a regular time that they fall asleep.

- Preference for evening hours. Many older children prefer being up later in the evening and at night, but school hours make it difficult for them to indulge this preference without depriving them of sleep.

- Bad sleep habits. Older children are more likely to have irregular schedules, to stay up late talking on the phone or playing on the computer, and drinking or eating caffeine, which interferes with the sleep-wake cycle.

- Narcolepsy, a rare neurological disorder that results in severe daytime sleepiness (the main symptom). Poor sleep, vivid dreams, and sleep paralysis are all symptoms of narcolepsy as is the telltale sign of falling asleep during normal daytime activities.

- Restless legs syndrome, a disorder that causes an uncomfortable feeling in the legs, causing the child to toss and turn and have difficulty falling asleep.

Good Sleep Habits

Developing good sleep habits can help address some of these problems. Others may require help from a physician or sleep specialist. To develop good sleep habits, work with your child to …

- Create a sleep plan.
- Follow it for two weeks.
- Keep a sleep log or ask your child to.
- Analyze your progress after 2 weeks.

The sleep plan should include strategies that the child agrees to follow to try to help improve his sleep. For example …

- Limiting TV and other stimulating activities in the hour or two before bedtime
- Keeping wake and sleep times consistent during the week and on the weekend
- Avoiding caffeine, especially in the evening

◆ Refraining from eating or drinking just before bed, as digestion can interfere with sleep. If hungry, a light snack can quell the pangs and help sleep.

◆ Practicing relaxation techniques

◆ Using the bed only for sleeping, not for reading, playing games, watching TV, or doing homework

◆ Signaling the daytime with open curtains and bright light

◆ Signaling nighttime by keeping the room quiet and dark and keeping exposure to bright light at a minimum during the evening hours

◆ Not exercising close to bedtime

> **Infant Almanac**
>
> An older child having trouble falling asleep should be allowed to get out of bed and read quietly or write in a journal until she feels sleepy. She shouldn't listen to music or watch TV, as this will interfere with her ability to fall asleep.
>
> Children at this age may also have nightmares and sleepwalking, common concerns that we discuss in Chapter 17.

Your child can also keep a sleep log to help identify potential problems.

Child's Sleep Log

My name: _____ Date: _____

I had _____ (number of) drinks with caffeine today.

What I did in the hour before bedtime (i.e., read a book, watched television, played on the computer): _____

_____

Did I have trouble falling asleep? _____

Did I wake up in the middle of the night? Why? _____

_____

How long did I sleep? _____

How much energy did I have today? _____

Did I pay attention in school today? _____

Did I take a nap today? _____

Encourage your child to look at the activities he did on the nights when he slept well. Remind him that when he gets more sleep, he has more energy the next day. Discuss other results so that he can learn how to develop better sleep habits based on the habits he describes.

Underlying Medical or Psychological Conditions

Certain medical conditions may also disrupt your older child's sleep. See Chapter 17 for a list of these conditions. In addition, difficulty sleeping may indicate the following:

♦ Psychological or behavioral problems, such as depression, anxiety disorder, or substance abuse

Infant Almanac

The onset of menstruation or a heavy period can cause some girls to have excessive fatigue during the day. The problem may not in fact be related to sleep habits. A visit to a gynecologist may be in order.

♦ School problems—not wanting to go to school because of lack of academic success, bullying, or other issues

♦ A medical problem interfering with sleep

♦ Medications for other disorders (such as epilepsy) interfering with sleep

Night Owl or Delayed Sleep Phase Syndrome?

Older children may show a preference for evening hours, but can go to sleep at a reasonable bedtime. Children with delayed sleep phase syndrome have an internal clock set differently from the rest of the world, which means they *can't* go to sleep earlier. Asking a child with delayed sleep phase syndrome to go to bed at a typical school-night bedtime is like asking an adult to go to bed at 6 P.M. You wouldn't fall asleep, either.

Children with delayed sleep phase syndrome can be treated. The hitch—you knew there'd be one, didn't you?—is that they have to be willing to participate in the plan.

Delayed sleep phase syndrome is treated by shifting the child's internal clock so that it coincides a little more closely with the rest of the world's. But be aware that shifting an internal clock isn't easy—you have to be committed and stick to it.

> **Infant Almanac**
>
> Delayed sleep phase syndrome is common in adolescents, but it affects younger children as well. However, before assuming that your child has delayed sleep phase syndrome, recognize that it's more likely she's just a night owl and prefers later hours. Either way, it's important to come up with a plan to make sure your child is getting an adequate amount of sleep.

The most common way to accomplish this is to shift the child's bedtime 15 minutes earlier each night until the child is going to bed at a reasonable bedtime.

However, shifting a bedtime earlier isn't always the best approach to treating delayed sleep phase syndrome. Just as it's more difficult to travel from east to west (going backward in time) than to travel west to east (going forward in time), it can also be very difficult to change an internal clock by advancing bedtime every night. Sleep clinicians find it more effective to delay bedtimes instead

This takes a bit more commitment because it requires that the child be allowed to sleep at different times throughout the day for at least a week in order to get to his target bedtime.

Here's how it works:

- ◆ On the first night, the child goes to bed at her regular bedtime (say, 2 A.M.) and is allowed to sleep until she wakes up naturally.

- ◆ On the next night, the child goes to bed at 5 A.M. and is allowed to sleep until she wakes up naturally.

- ◆ This process continues in 3-hour increments until the child is going to bed at 9 P.M. (or the target bedtime).

- ◆ The new bedtime is maintained strictly. It becomes the new "set point."

Often this is an unrealistic solution since children need to get up and go to school, but it is generally more effective than trying to make the child go to bed earlier. You may be able to time the process for a school break or vacation.

Choosing the Most Effective Method for Your Older Child

As is the case for younger children, for older children you will need to be firm in helping them to establish or maintain good sleep hygiene (good sleep habits).

This can be particularly difficult, as children this age are becoming more and more independent (at least until they need something) and are starting to shun their parents' wisdom. What's a parent to do?

Parents of older children can talk to them about the importance of sleep in functioning well during the day. Now that your child can think logically (at least in theory), it is possible to discuss good sleep habits with her, emphasizing that it's what her body needs (just like good nutrition).

Infant Almanac

There are several websites designed for children that discuss the importance of sleep. Links can be found on the National Sleep Foundation website (www.sleepfoundation.org).

Sleep is a relatively cool subject and your older child may be more willing to listen to you or read about sleep than, say, world history, so don't give up before you try to have a conversation or two (or ten) with your child.

Keep in mind that to treat some sleep disorders in older children, you will need the help of a sleep specialist. Just as it's difficult for adults to solve their own sleep problems, it will be more difficult to try to solve your older child's. Sleep training an older child is no longer a matter of leaving the room, closing the door, and putting on a set of headphones while the baby cries. You do that with an older child and he'll just switch on the TV, cell phone, iPod ... you get the picture.

If your child has established a good bedtime routine and you have done all you can to help her establish good sleep hygiene, yet she still shows signs of having a sleep problem, then it's time to see a sleep specialist.

The Least You Need to Know

♦ Some older children *can't* go to bed at a reasonable hour—they have delayed sleep phase syndrome, which naturally occurs among many children as they enter puberty.

♦ Older children can have realistic, though usually groundless, fears that can keep them awake.

♦ Most older children don't get enough sleep.

♦ Bad sleep habits can be changed with a plan and some effort.

Chapter 19

Helping Children with Special Needs Sleep Soundly

In This Chapter

- ◆ Coping with sleep problems common to children with special needs
- ◆ Dealing with sleep problems caused by medications
- ◆ Recognizing how sleep problems can influence medical or psychological problems
- ◆ Seeking help for sleep problems in children with special needs

As if children with special needs (and their parents) didn't have enough to cope with, they're more likely than other children to have sleep problems.

In this chapter, we'll discuss how children with special needs end up with more sleep problems, and we'll give you information on how to handle those problems. We'll also describe when it's time to call in the sleep specialists to help you deal with the sleep difficulties facing you and your child.

Special Considerations for Children with Special Needs

Children with special needs of any type (physical, mental, emotional) are more prone to sleep difficulties than other children. They have trouble falling asleep and staying asleep, and they're more likely to have restless sleep, which means that their sleep is not as restorative for them as it should be.

Trouble sleeping makes your child with special needs (and you!) even less able to deal with the difficulties caused by his special needs.

For example, a child with asthma might wheeze throughout the night, disrupting sleep. In fact, a recent poll found that 48 percent of children with asthma had disrupted sleep. As with other children, disrupted nighttime sleep can lead to daytime behavior problems and sleepiness.

So making sure everyone gets a good sleep should be a priority for you and your child with special needs. But you should be aware of some special challenges you'll face:

- ◆ Your child may take longer to develop good sleep habits.
- ◆ She may resist the changes you implement.
- ◆ She may not completely understand your motives.

Common Sleep Problems of Children with Special Needs

Children with special needs are more likely to have trouble sleeping for these reasons:

- ◆ Physical pain because of their medical problem may disrupt sleep.
- ◆ Symptoms of the medical problem (e.g., wheezing in a child with asthma) may disrupt sleep.

◆ Medications used to treat the problem (e.g., antidepressants and antianxiety drugs) can cause sleep problems.

◆ A child on medication for a problem might experience sleep disruption because of a *paradoxical effect* of the medication itself.

Children with special needs also suffer from sleep disruptions caused by nightmares and night terrors, and may also sleepwalk and sleep talk. See Chapter 17 for more information about these problems. You may want to seek a specialist's advice for dealing with these problems in a child with special needs.

> **Infant Almanac**
>
> Medication used to treat various problems in children can not only increase sleep problems, but can also increase daytime sleepiness, resulting in more difficulties for the child.

> **BABY BABBLE**
>
> A **paradoxical effect** is one that is opposite to the reaction intended. It's a term generally used to refer to a medication that does the opposite of what it is supposed to do—for example, a sedative that induces hyperactive behavior in some children.

Effect of Sleep Problems in Children with Special Needs

Children with special needs who have sleep problems also frequently experience an increase in physical and mental health difficulties. Sleep problems lead to …

◆ Decreased coping skills.

◆ Increased levels of frustration.

◆ Less self-control.

◆ Decreased compliance with treatment.

◆ Increased aggression.

◆ Increased self-injury behaviors.

◆ Increased stress on an already stressed family.

Steps to Take

Clearly, the first thing to do is control, as much as possible, symptoms of the child's medical problems that interfere with sleep. For example, improving a child with asthma's treatment and preventing asthma attacks at night will reduce sleep disruptions. In a child with epilepsy, efforts to improve night-time control of seizures can improve the quality of sleep that the child experiences. In the same way, finding appropriate pain-relieving medications will help the child with a painful physical problem sleep more easily at night.

In addition, changing the child's medication (in consultation with the child's doctors, of course!) may help improve the child's sleep.

> **Infant Almanac**
>
> Don't overlook the fact that your child with special needs could have another medical condition, such as sleep apnea (breathing cessation), that contributes to his sleeping difficulties. A thorough evaluation can help reassure you that you're doing everything you can to help your child sleep.

Encouraging the child with special needs to get adequate rest may include earlier bedtimes than might be expected in a child without difficulties or perhaps later wake times in the morning (depending on the child).

Keeping the child from becoming overstimulated and overtired also improves her chances of getting a good night's sleep. Many children with special needs are especially susceptible to disturbances caused by light and noise, so reducing these can improve sleep. A white noise machine may help the child who is overly sensitive to the sound of the dog's nails on the carpet. An autistic child may be very sensitive to the way his pajamas and bedding feel. Work with your child to come up with the most comfortable environment for him to sleep in.

Developing a set schedule and a bedtime routine is very reassuring for children with special needs—perhaps even more so than for other children. In most cases, being consistent and firm with bedtimes helps children with special needs get the sleep they need. Try the following:

◆ Let your child know what happens next. Create a chart of the bedtime routine with pictures so that your child can know what to expect every evening.

◆ Focus on relaxing activities before bed. For some children with special needs, a bath might be soothing; for others, it's a source of agitation and shouldn't be attempted just before bedtime.

◆ Build in repetition. Read the same book each night (until your child requests a different one); follow the bedtime routine in the same sequence of events every night.

Infant Almanac

Medications to help encourage sleep are usually not the best choice for children with special needs. Not only may sleep medications interfere with other medications the child may be taking, but there is also evidence that sleep medications can actually increase sleep problems in children, especially those with special needs.

Hospitalization

Any child can end up in the hospital needing an emergency appendectomy, and this experience may disrupt their sleep, create stress, and cause some anxiety afterward. Children with special needs are more likely to be hospitalized frequently.

Frequent hospitalizations are incredibly stressful and disruptive for a child (and her family).

If your child is hospitalized, you can try to reduce the disruption by doing the following:

◆ Follow the bedtime routine you follow at home (as much as possible).

◆ Bring your child's own pajamas and a favorite toy, blanket, or lovey.

◆ Bring pictures of family members.

◆ Create a special, relaxing routine for bedtime.

◆ Decide whether to sleep in the hospital room based on your child's needs, not yours. Some children find their parent's presence disruptive, whereas others find it more comforting to have you in the room.

◆ Ask that painful procedures not be performed in the bed so the child does not associate it with needles and catheters.

◆ Return to normal as soon as you can.

Attention Deficit-Hyperactivity Disorder (ADHD)

ADHD is the most common psychiatric disorder among children. Common symptoms include difficulty paying attention, distractibility, difficulty in transitioning from one task to another, and lack of impulse control. Older children may have trouble with being organized and with complex thinking tasks.

If this sounds a lot like a sleep-deprived child, you're right. That's why some children with sleep problems are incorrectly diagnosed with ADHD. Sometimes, solving the sleep disturbances can eliminate all symptoms of ADHD.

On the other hand, some children with ADHD experience disturbed sleep, and the symptoms of ADHD do not go away by helping the child sleep better. In either case, helping the child with his sleep issues will at least help improve some symptoms.

> **Infant Almanac**
>
> The side effects of ADHD medications, especially stimulants like Ritalin, cause problems falling asleep. Also, as the medication wears off at the end of the day, ADHD symptoms may increase, making sleep more difficult.

Just like any other child, your child may also have difficulty sleeping because of the following:

◆ Sleep associations (needing a parent to be present to fall asleep)

◆ Anxieties

◆ Poor sleep habits

You may want to follow these strategies to help resolve the problem:

◆ Check your child's medications. An adjustment to the medication dosage, type of medication, or combination of medications may make all the difference.

◆ Treat medical, behavior, and psychiatric problems.

♦ Do what works—strategies that are effective in other children may work for your child with ADHD.

♦ Try a reward system.

♦ Encourage good sleep habits.

♦ Maintain a calm environment.

Neurological Problems, Autism, and Severe Developmental Delays

In children with neurological problems, sleep problems may actually be caused by faulty "wiring" in the brain. Children with these problems are also less able to deal with difficulties caused by poor sleep. Even worse, sleep deprivation in children with developmental delays and other neurological problems may cause self-injurious and aggressive behavior.

Children with severe developmental delays are particularly prone to sleep problems. Studies have shown that almost all children with autism have sleep difficulties, and that 80 percent of children with developmental delays have trouble sleeping (with 25 percent of these being characterized as "severe").

However, these sleep problems may be treatable. Don't just assume that the sleep difficulty is part of the "problem" (your child's disorder) and must be suffered through. Seek help from your child's pediatrician or neurologist. It may be necessary to see a sleep specialist in order to treat the sleep disorder.

BABY BABBLE

Autism is a developmental disability that usually appears before age 3. The result of a neurological disorder that disrupts normal functions in the brain, it delays and alters social and communication skills.

Infant Almanac

Unlike typically developing children, children with special needs often do not outgrow their sleep problems. Consulting with a sleep specialist early on can save a lot of wear and tear on your nerves.

Solving Sleep Problems in Children with Special Needs

Many of the same techniques that work with other children work with children with special needs. For example, try the following techniques:

- Maintain good sleep habits.

- Keep set wake and sleep hours (when possible).

- Create positive sleep associations (so that you don't have to be present for your child to fall asleep).

- Allow an extra-long transition period before bedtime.

- Take care of stressful stuff (homework) well before bedtime.

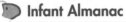 **Infant Almanac**

The most important thing to remember is to be patient. Children with special needs will likely require longer for sleep-training methods to work.

In addition, make sure you're treating and controlling symptoms of the problem that might disrupt sleep. For example, if your child has allergies that disrupt her sleep, control the symptoms with medication and keep her bedroom as allergen-free as possible.

Getting Help for Children with Special Needs

Some sleep-training approaches work better than others for helping children with special needs get a good night's rest.

Some parents, for example, have found that the "scheduled awakenings" approach (see Chapter 10) has worked particularly well for their autistic children. But this might not be the right approach for a child with a different problem.

If your child with special needs has difficulty getting enough rest, and the strategies suggested here don't work, consult your pediatrician. Your child may also benefit from a visit with a specialist or even a visit to a sleep center.

Since many pediatricians don't receive much training in treating sleep problems, it's wise for parents seeking help to find a pediatric sleep specialist (a Ph.D or an M.D.) for a thorough assessment. Sleep specialists have been trained and know how to properly diagnose and treat sleep disorders.

Some sleep disorders, such as sleep apnea, require a sleep study in order to be diagnosed. A sleep study involves the child's sleep being assessed by measuring brain waves, muscle tone, leg movement, breathing, and heart rate during sleep. Sometimes such a study can be done at home, but more often it requires an overnight visit to a sleep clinic. The benefits of a good diagnosis outweigh the inconveniences the sleep study may cause.

> **Unhappy Baby Alert**
>
> Parents of children with special needs are often sleep-deprived themselves. Don't forget to ask for help and to seek the advice of a physician for yourself! And take a glance at Chapter 5 for some ideas on how to get a little rest.

> **Melissa's Mindset**
>
> One good book that deals specifically with sleep problems in children with special needs is *Sleep Better! A Guide to Improving Sleep for Children with Special Needs*, by Mark Durand, Ph.D.

The Least You Need to Know

- Children with special needs are prone to sleep difficulties.

- Many of the same approaches that work for other children will work for children with special needs.

- Medications for many medical, behavioral (ADHD), and emotional (depression) problems can cause sleep disruptions.

- Many sleep problems in children with special needs are treatable.

5

Holistic and New Age Methods

If you deal with stress by finding a quiet corner and meditating, we've got some great information for you!

In this part, we'll share ideas for using yoga, massage, and music to help lull your baby to sleep. You can use many of these methods in addition to other sleep-training methods to help prepare your baby to fall asleep.

Chapter

20

You Are Getting Sleepy: Using Hypnosis, Meditation, and Other Mental Strategies

In This Chapter

◆ Understanding how hypnosis and self-hypnosis work

◆ Using the power of the mind (your child's mind) to encourage relaxation and sleep

◆ Showing your child how meditation can help her calm down and settle for bed

◆ How positive thoughts (affirmations) can help create good sleep habits

In this chapter, we'll focus on the power of the mind to help your child learn to relax and fall asleep. The techniques we describe in this chapter may seem a little New Age-y, but they work! We'll explain how—and show you why you should think about using them to help your child relax and get ready for bed.

The Power of the Mind

Your mind is a powerful instrument—and so is your child's. But we don't often think about how we can use our minds, or encourage our children to use *theirs*, in order to ensure a peaceful night's sleep.

But for your young child (one who is able, at least, to understand and follow directions), harnessing the power of the mind to help her relax and settle for bed helps put her in control. Once she learns the techniques, they're hers for life. She'll be able to use them whenever she faces challenges or stresses—and when she has a preschooler of her own who resists bedtime!

In this Part, we talk about some New Age-y activities, like meditation, yoga (see Chapter 21), and Feng Shui (see Chapter 22). All of these activities can be enhanced by focusing the power of the mind on what you (or in this case, your child) want to accomplish.

The Power of Affirmations

BABY BABBLE

Affirmations are positive thoughts you can teach your child to think as he meditates, such as "I do well in school," or "I have good friends and am a good friend." The idea is that instead of listening to the negative, stressful thoughts in his brain, he can create positive affirmations to replace them.

When you're showing your child how to meditate or when you use Feng Shui to create a soothing environment for your child (see Chapter 22), you increase your chances of success if you use the power of *affirmations*.

When your child sits down to meditate, have him think an affirmation as he does so: "I am relaxed and ready for the rest I need."

The Power of Intentions

An intention, simply put, is the reason you're doing what you're doing. By setting your alarm, you're intending to get up in time for work.

Children understand the power of intentions quite well, especially if you explain how they work.

You can harvest the power of intentions during meditation and while doing other activities. For example, when you sit down to meditate with your child, not only can you have her start with an affirmation (such as, "I am at peace with the world") but also with an intention that explains why she's doing what she's doing: "By meditating, I calm myself and let the stresses of the day go away."

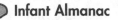 **Infant Almanac**

Your child can also use affirmations throughout the day to help deal with stresses and to keep strong emotions, like anger, in check. For instance, if someone teases him about his small stature, he can say, to himself: "I am big in courage and confidence."

Brainstorm some intentions with your child to use as you practice the activities in this Part (Chapters 20, 21, and 22).

Using Hypnosis to Help Your Little One Sleep

Self-hypnosis, a method of creating focused concentration in your mind, can also be a method you can use to learn to relax your body. This helps sleep come more easily. Self-hypnosis techniques can be taught even to a young child to help her relax and fall asleep. Hypnosis itself isn't sleep, it's just a way to help bring about sleep. You can do the technique at any time throughout the day, though close to bedtime may be most realistic since it's easiest for your child to enter the hypnotic state by sitting or lying down and relaxing.

Infant Almanac

You can't use hypnosis or teach self-hypnosis to infants, but if your child can understand simple commands, he can learn the techniques—though you'll have to help him at first.

The core of hypnosis is induction, the process of entering the hypnotic state. A ritual that helps create the transition is usually followed. In most cases, this ritual includes progressive physical relaxation.

Melissa's Mindset

Although there has been no research conducted that specifically looks at the impact of hypnosis on sleep in children, some adult research has shown that hypnosis can be effective for treating some forms of sleep disorder. There's no indication that hypnosis is dangerous for children, so if it sounds like something you'd like to try with your child, go for it! But keep in mind that if these techniques do not seem to help, you should consult a sleep specialist.

Achieving Progressive Muscle Relaxation (PMR)

Starting with your head, you work your way down to your toes, relaxing each set of muscles as you go.

To teach your child self-hypnosis, you'll cue her by using a soft, even tone and saying, "Relax your face … close your eyes … now relax your jaw … relax your neck." You can gently touch the part to be relaxed as you speak. Use a slow, soft, soothing voice.

If your child has difficulty relaxing the body part, have him tense it first. This gives him a physical reminder of where that body part is and how to relax it. So to relax his hand, he might make a tight fist and then loosen his hand until it's totally relaxed.

Once he's completely relaxed, guide him to a peaceful place (imaginary or real) where he feels happy and relaxed. Ask him to tell you about the place. It is important to have the child use all of her senses to really make the place real. For example, encourage her to smell the ocean, taste the ice cream, and feel the sun on her skin or the sand between her toes. Then, still using a soft, soothing voice, introduce sleep suggestions, such as the following:

Infant Almanac

The hypnosis session will always end no matter what; no one stays in the hypnotic state for very long. The important thing is to show your child how to enter the state.

♦ "You will fall asleep quickly and stay asleep until morning."

♦ "If you need to awaken at night, such as to use the bathroom, you will quickly fall asleep as soon as you go back to bed."

♦ "When you wake up, you will feel happy and rested."

◆ "You won't let sounds or other
disturbances bother you during
the night."

After a few minutes, gently tell your
child that the session has ended and
he can get up when he's ready.

Once your child is able to enter the
hypnotic state under your guidance,
you can encourage him to do it him-
self. He will progressively relax as you've shown him how. He may want
to hold a small object in his hand. As soon as he's relaxed enough to let
go of the small object, he has entered the hypnotic state.

After he feels totally relaxed, he can visualize the outcome he wants to
achieve—for example, he can visualize himself closing his eyes and falling asleep easily and without tossing and turning; he can visualize himself having good dreams and waking
in the morning feeling energetic and
rested.

A few minutes later he will "wake up"
from the hypnotic state. He can also
use a timer or alarm that doesn't jar
him, to help arouse him from the state.

You can also use music to help relax
a child during a self-hypnosis session. See Chapter 22 for more information.

Unhappy Baby Alert

Don't give up if your
first few attempts at hypnosis don't reduce the wiggles
in your preschooler. Hypnosis
and self-hypnosis are techniques that improve with practice! Keep at it and eventually
your child will respond.

Infant Almanac

Researchers at the
University of Michigan
say there's some evidence from
individual case studies that
teaching children self-hypnosis
can also help them cope with
habits and tics, such as thumb-
sucking and hair-pulling; bedwetting, sleep terrors, and other
sleep disturbances; as well as
anxiety and stress.

Making Nightmares Go Away

You and your child can use hypnosis to help make scary dreams and
nightmares disappear. Follow these guidelines:

◆ First, at some time during the day (not right at bedtime), discuss
the nightmare with your child. Find out what happens in the
nightmare (or the types of things that happen in the nightmares
she has, if it's not a recurring dream).

- Then, with your child, create an alternative scenario to what happens in the nightmare. For example, perhaps a hero (whom you carefully discuss and describe) saves the day; or perhaps the scary monster turns out to be kind-hearted; or your child finds a way to turn something scary into something fun and exciting.

- Have your child close her eyes and rehearse what to do in her nightmares to turn them into good dreams.

- Now, at bedtime, have your child enter the hypnotic state, as described earlier.

Melissa's Mindset

Portions of this technique can be used without full hypnosis. Children can be helped to realize they can control their dreams by thinking positive thoughts before bedtime and getting out of dreams—or even changing them—when they are too scary.

- Then tell her that her old nightmares are gone, replaced with this new scenario. If she has a nightmare, she will wake up before it gets too scary and it will go away.

- Let your child gradually come out of the hypnotic state.

- When she falls asleep, she should have fewer—or no—nightmares.

Finding a Hypnotherapist

To get started with self-hypnosis for your child, you may want to work with a hypnotherapist, at least for a session or two.

Pediatric hypnotherapists teach children how to self-hypnotize and can show you how to help your child with the method. However, be aware that anyone can hang up a shingle and call himself a "hypnotherapist," so you'll want to look for one who's certified by the American Society of Clinical Hypnosis.

Omm ... How Meditation Can Help Your Child Sleep

Another relaxation technique, meditation, can help children relax enough to fall asleep. Meditation can be particularly helpful for anxious children or those who are dealing with stress from school or personal life.

Although there are many variations, essentially meditation involves clearing the mind of all the thoughts that clutter it up. In this case, the purpose would be to relax so that it's easy to fall asleep at bedtime.

Starting Meditation

To help your child learn the basics of meditation, you'll have to be a role model. Sit with him quietly for a few minutes just before bedtime, with no talking and eyes closed. Gradually lengthen the amount of time you sit quietly with no talking and eyes closed.

For sitting meditation, do the following:

- ◆ Sit cross-legged on the ground.

- ◆ Let your hands rest lightly on your legs.

- ◆ Keep your body straight and relaxed.

- ◆ Tuck your pelvis under slightly.

- ◆ If you need back support, you may sit in a chair.

- ◆ Focus on your breathing: feel the air entering and leaving your body.

Next, work on breathing slowly in and out. By consciously slowing his breath, he'll relax. Once he's breathing slowly, have him relax his muscles. As he exhales, tell him that all the unhappy or unpleasant thoughts, cares, and concerns are leaving his body. As he inhales, he is bringing in good, positive energy to help him sleep. He should focus on the breath coming into and leaving his body.

Infant Almanac

If it coincides with your religious beliefs, teach your child to say prayers as a prelude to meditation. Saying prayers before bed can help your child relax and feel safe and secure.

Then, introduce the idea of clearing the mind by focusing on a peaceful, pleasant image. This is usually a place that the child has been to or imagines. He mentally walks around the place, thinking of everything he likes about the place.

A younger child may want to tell you all about it, but encourage him to keep his thoughts in his head and to focus on how happy and relaxed he feels when he is at this peaceful place.

Using Guided Imagery

You can also guide your child in her imagery. For example, show her pictures of the ocean (or if she has been to the ocean, remind her what it looks like). Then, at meditation time, have your child think about the ocean, the waves going in and out, the sand on the beach, the warm sun relaxing her muscles. This guided imagery can help a child learn how to empty her mind of stressful and negative thoughts, making it easier for her to fall asleep.

If your child is having difficulty focusing even with guided imagery, have her think of a mantra or repetitive phrase that she can use to focus her mind. It could be a nonsense word or an affirmation such as "I feel joyful."

Infant Almanac

Children as young as 5 can practice meditation to help them sleep.

Because children can get stressed throughout the day, learning how to take a few minutes to calm down through meditation can lower their stress levels and ultimately reduce their sleep problems.

Melissa's Mindset

As with hypnosis, there is no research looking at the effects of meditation on sleep in children. But for children with anxiety or who have trouble winding down at bedtime, adding meditation to a bedtime routine could certainly help. Meditation may also be used in conjunction with more conventional approaches to treating sleep or other problems in children, rather than as a "treatment" in and of itself. Some clinicians find that adding meditation to a child's treatment plan can help lessen pain and anxiety.

Wiggly kids who can't stay still long enough to meditate may benefit from walking meditation. This approach enables them to engage their bodies while clearing their minds. Go for a walk with your child, and encourage him to focus on moving slowly, feeling his left leg as it moves, and then his right leg. By being quiet and focusing on his body, he can clear his mind and feel refreshed and relaxed, even if he can't sit still long enough to do guided imagery with you.

The Least You Need to Know

- ◆ Affirmations and intentions can help your child feel more positive and less stressed.

- ◆ Hypnosis can help your child sleep by showing her how to relax and by introducing suggestions into her mind that will help her sleep.

- ◆ An older child can use self-hypnosis to sleep better.

- ◆ Hypnosis can help eliminate nightmares.

- ◆ Meditation can help children relax and de-stress before bed.

Chapter 21

The Sleeping Child Pose: Using Yoga, Massage, and Other Physical Techniques

In This Chapter

- Understanding how physical techniques can help soothe and relax your child and help him prepare for bedtime
- Using massage to relax your child and help you connect with her
- How swaddling can help calm overstimulated babies
- Performing yoga and Tai Chi to de-stress and settle down

In this chapter, we'll focus on the power of the body—doing physical movements—to help your child relax and feel ready for bedtime. We'll explain how teaching your child elements of yoga and Tai Chi can help him ease stress and tension and get ready for bed.

And we'll show you how you can use massage and swaddling on your child to help him feel nurtured and relaxed—also with the intention of helping him sleep. These methods can become part of your bedtime ritual.

A Breath of Fresh Air

Physical exercises such as Tai Chi and yoga and mental exercises such as meditation (see Chapter 20) emphasize the importance of breathing properly. Since your child has been breathing all her life, you may wonder why you have to teach her.

> **Infant Almanac**
>
> Your child can use conscious breathing to help his meditation, yoga, and/or Tai Chi exercises. Doing so increases the relaxation these exercises bring and can help him de-stress in preparation for sleep.

The simplest thing you can do is to have your child breathe deeply in through the nose and out through the mouth. This also helps relax the jaw and face muscles. Show your child how to put her hands on her abdomen so that she can feel the air coming into her body. Like adults, children often breathe shallowly, which increases stress and tension. Deeper breaths can help relieve tension.

Have your child place her hands on her abdomen as she inhales to feel it expand as she breathes. Encourage her to make herself "fat" with air.

Then, have your child slowly lengthen the amount of time she takes to draw the breath in and let it out. Start with 3 seconds to inhale and 3 seconds to exhale and build to 10 seconds for each. Consciously slowing her breathing will help her relax and clear her mind.

Melissa's Mindset

Taking deep breaths can help children learn to de-stress throughout the day, not just at bedtime. When Jennifer's daughter was in pre-school, she would get easily agitated when she had to transition from one task to another or when she couldn't say what she wanted. Jennifer taught her how to "take a deep breath" and soon Jessica would remember to do that whenever her anxiety grew. It helped her relax and calm down, and it made it easier for her to express her needs. Her teachers marveled at how much difference this made with her behavior and soon started teaching all the other students! I use the same technique with my son Nickolas.

Child/Family Yoga

Yoga is an Eastern practice that encourages health and well-being. Practitioners move their bodies into various "poses" that help stretch the body, work joints, and stimulate muscles.

You can show your child *restorative poses* to help him relax, as opposed to active yoga techniques that ramp energy up.

Yoga can be done with infants—the parent does some exercises with the baby to build muscle awareness and to enjoy interacting with the baby. Two- and three-year-olds are more independent and can do kid-level yoga exercises with some direction from parents or a yoga teacher. Older children can do more sophisticated exercises and need less supervision.

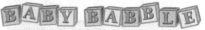

Restorative poses are calm yoga poses that soothe body and mind. Many people use yoga poses to help them meditate. Use supported, relaxing poses to encourage your child to relax and let go.

Infant Yoga

When your child is a baby, you can do some simple stretches to introduce him to yoga. These are easy, unforced stretches that enable you and your baby to exchange the bond of touching and can help settle the baby for bedtime.

One simple stretch is to bring the baby's arms together over his chest, and then gently pull them apart, like wings. You can also gently stretch baby's arms over his head and back down again.

Melissa's Mindset

Incidentally, the leg-stretching pose can help a baby with gastrointestinal pain or constipation as well!

You can gently cycle your baby's legs, as if she were riding a bike. A leg-stretching pose can be done by pushing the leg, in a bent-knee position, toward your baby's torso, and then gently stretching it back down.

Relaxing Yoga Poses for Children Young and Old

Your young child (age 2 or 3) can start doing some yoga poses with your help. As he gets older he may need less supervision, but you may still want to join him for some quality time together.

Melissa's Mindset

In Nickolas' preschool, a yoga teacher comes in weekly to work with the 1-, 2-, 3-, and 4-year-old children. Although when Nickolas was younger, he often would not actively participate, he knew the poses and would practice them at home. Now he looks forward to yoga days and comes home with moves he teaches me!

Your child will feel the effect of the poses right away. If he prefers some over others, that's fine. Let him choose the poses that make him feel best.

Modified Lotus Pose

This pose stretches muscles and relaxes the body. Start with 1 or 2 minutes and build up to 5 minutes.

1. Sit with your back against a wall.

2. Place the soles of your feet together.

3. Put a folded towel or blanket under each knee to prop it up.

4. Rest your hands on your knees.

5. Sit up straight with back, neck, and head aligned.

6. Close eyes and breathe.

Forward Bend

This pose stretches muscles and relaxes the body. Start with 1 or 2 minutes and build to 5 minutes.

1. Sit with legs stretched out in front of you.

2. Keep back straight and shoulders back.

3. Bend your chest down toward your knees. Stop when you feel a pull—don't stretch too much as you may hurt yourself.

4. Hold while closing eyes and breathing.

Wall Pose

This pose stretches muscles and relaxes the body. Start with 1 or 2 minutes and build to 5 minutes.

1. Lie on your back with your knees pulled up to your chest, so that your body is perpendicular to a wall and your buttocks are touching or close to touching the wall. Place a folded towel in the small of your back if needed for support.

2. Extend your legs up the wall so they rest against the wall.

3. Adjust your body so that the position can be maintained comfortably.

4. Stretch your arms over your head comfortably, with no strain. They should rest on the floor behind you.

5. Close your eyes and breathe.

Unhappy Baby Alert

If your child has any difficulty with any of the poses, don't force the issue. If the poses your child prefers change from day to day, that's all right, too.

Child's Pose

This pose stretches muscles and helps the child feel relaxed and supported. Start with 1 or 2 minutes in the pose and build to 5 minutes.

1. Kneel on the floor, feet together.

2. Place a folded towel or blanket across your legs. The towel will support your chest as you bend at the waist, so stack as many as needed to help you feel comfortable and supported.

3. Bending forward, rest your chest on the towel(s). Turn your head to one side. After a minute, turn your head to the other side.

4. Relax arms comfortably to either side of you.

5. Close your eyes and breathe slowly and calmly.

Resting Pose

This pose encourages supported relaxation. You can also use it to encourage visualization or meditation in your child. Start with 1 or 2 minutes and build up to 5 minutes.

> **Infant Almanac**
>
> Have your child think of a peaceful scene while she's doing the poses, and make sure she moves slowly from one pose to the next. Challenge her to move like a turtle instead of a rabbit.

1. Lie on your back with a rolled towel beneath your knees and a folded blanket under your head.

2. Spread your arms out in a comfortable position.

3. If you need more support, place folded blankets or towels under wrists and ankles.

4. Close eyes and breathe deeply.

Tai Chi and Your Child

Like yoga, Tai Chi exercises can help your child relax and feel ready for sleep.

Tai Chi (or Taiji), meaning "Grand Ultimate Fist," is an ancient Chinese martial art that is based on Taoist philosophy. Tai Chi encourages a supple, flexible mind, body, and spirit.

Tai Chi consists of slow, connected movements that help your chi (life energy) to circulate freely. Traditional Chinese medicine authorities believe that blocked chi causes mental and physical illness. By doing the exercises, you open up the channels that chi energy moves through.

Basic Tai Chi Exercises

Some basic exercises can help your child relax and get rid of stress. You may want to do the exercises with your child at first until he can do them on his own.

Open and Close Heaven and Earth

This exercise helps collect energy from nature and dispel negative energy.

1. Stand with feet about one-and-a-half shoulders' width apart, knees slightly bent.

2. Create a circle with your hands, as if you were hugging a tree. Cup your palms.

3. Raise your arms up until they're fully extended above your head.

4. Rotate your wrists away from your body so that your palms face the sky.

5. Slowly lower your arms to your sides.

6. Repeat.

> **Infant Almanac**
>
> Your child can also meditate while doing the exercises. This is particularly good for children who have trouble sitting still.

Lower Chi and Cleanse Internally

This exercise helps collect energy from nature and dispel negative energy.

1. Stand in a relaxed posture with your feet comfortably apart and your arms hanging at your side.

2. Straighten your body so you're standing tall and bring your arms above your head.

3. At the same time, breathe in. Visualize that you're collecting energy from nature.

4. Visualize bringing the energy into your head and down through your body. Visualize letting the negative energy come out of your body from your feet.

5. Repeat.

Finding a Tai Chi Instructor

You may want to find a Tai Chi instructor to help your child learn some of the movements. These guidelines will help:

- The teacher is more important than the style of Tai Chi (there are many different styles of Tai Chi, based on the same basic movements).

- Ask friends and colleagues for referrals.

- Investigate all the resources in your area—clubs, parks and recreation programs, commercial schools.

- Meet the teacher and watch a few classes before signing up.

- Talk with the students about their experiences.

Swaddling Your New Baby

Swaddling is wrapping your baby in a blanket for warmth and security. Newborns especially can find swaddling soothing and it can calm them down enough to sleep. Swaddling the baby reminds her of being closely held, which feels good. Some people think it works because it reminds the newborn of being in the womb. Even if you don't swaddle your baby regularly, it can help under certain circumstances, such as when she's overstimulated.

Infant Almanac

Swaddling also helps if your baby is a restless sleeper and smacks himself in the face a lot. Wrapping him securely in a blanket will help prevent that.

Swaddling may also help colicky infants feel warm and secure, which may calm them and reduce the tears.

Wrap the baby from the shoulders down in a sheet or light receiving blanket. Your baby may prefer to be swaddled firmly so that hands and feet can't get loose; others like to be able to move their arms at least a little.

Follow these steps to swaddle your baby:

- Lay the sheet or receiving blanket out flat. Fold one corner over.

- Place your baby on his back on the sheet with the fold against his neck.

- Take the left corner of the sheet, draw it across his body, and tuck it under him.

- Pull the bottom corner up over his feet.

- Take the right corner of the sheet, draw it across his body and tuck it in.

- Don't cover the baby's head or neck.

- Don't use a heavy blanket. If your baby seems warm, loosen the swaddling or use a lighter weight sheet.

Massaging Your Infant or Child

Massage is using touch to stroke, rub, and manipulate the soft tissue of the body to relieve stress and promote health. Eastern thought is that tight muscles represent blocked energy. Unblocking the energy improves health and well-being.

Beyond this, touch is important to your child. You can use it to reassure your infant or child of your presence. A father can use massage to connect with a breastfeeding baby. A kind touch will help your child relax. Even a simple, no-frills back rub can help your child settle and feel more ready for bed.

As you're massaging your baby or child, listen to your intuition. Your child may not be able to tell you if a particular spot is tender or if she's extremely stressed. Use your intuition to guide you as you do the massage. Remember to always start with a light touch.

Melissa's Mindset

Some research has found that massage is helpful for high-risk infants (such as those born pre-term) especially. Some researchers find increases in weight gain and shorter hospital stays for pre-term infants who experience gentle massage.

Infant Almanac

Massage can make both the giver and the receiver feel good. Massage with an infant or child can help both of you connect and enjoy each other.

> **Infant Almanac**
>
> If you plan to go to a massage therapist, make sure she is certified as a massage therapist—look for a certification from a massage school. Some organizations, such as the National Certification Board for Therapeutic Massage and Bodywork, certify professionals who adhere to set standards and demonstrate competency. Ask friends and colleagues for a referral. Massage therapists often work with chiropractors, naturopaths, and acupuncturists.

When Not to Massage

Under certain circumstances, it's better not to give your baby or your child a massage. For example ...

♦ When your child is running a fever, a massage may interfere with the body's disease-fighting process. Ask your child's pediatrician if a massage will help.

♦ When your child has a sunburn, cuts, or a rash on his skin, a massage may aggravate the condition.

♦ If your child has a chronic condition, such as diabetes, check with his pediatrician before giving massages.

♦ If your child is in a lot pain, massage may not help. Discover the reason for the pain first.

♦ If your child has trouble breathing, such as during an asthma attack, don't give a massage.

♦ If your child is having a panic attack or extreme anxiety, let the attack pass first before giving a massage.

♦ If your child feels uncomfortable with your touch, stop.

♦ Don't massage your child's eyes.

♦ Don't massage your child when you're angry or frustrated with her—those emotions will be communicated through touch.

Getting Started

Always begin a massage session with the intention of healing. Never force yourself to give a massage and never make your child receive one. Follow these guidelines:

- ◆ Groom yourself. Make sure your hands are clean, your nails are trimmed, and your jewelry has been removed.

- ◆ Get comfortable. Both you and your child should feel relaxed and comfortable. Use blankets and pillows to support your child's body. You should wear something comfortable and easy to maneuver in. Cover your child with a blanket for warmth and security.

- ◆ Make the room comfortable. The temperature should be warm enough that bare skin doesn't get cold. Keep the lights low—though you should be able to see what you're doing.

- ◆ Get rid of distractions, noise, visual stimulation. Turn off the television, and close the door. Playing some soothing music may help everyone relax.

- ◆ You can use oil or lotion to reduce the friction as you massage and make it easier for you and more pleasant for your child. Oil is most slippery. Try jojoba oil, as it rarely causes an allergic reaction. You can also try lavender body lotion since lavender helps people relax.

- ◆ Encourage your child to breathe slowly and deeply to help her relax. You should do so, too.

Unhappy Baby Alert

You may want to avoid using essential oils on babies and children since the oils can be strong. Nut oils may trigger an allergy, so they should be avoided, too. Warm the oil or lotion in your hands first before placing it on your child's skin.

Massaging Your Infant

Infant massage encourages bonding with your child, and promotes mental, emotional, and physical health. Good touch equals safety and ove to your baby. Massage can help your overstimulated baby relax and get some sleep. Follow these guidelines:

- Always use a light touch.

- Give baby a chance to get accustomed to touch.

- Use light strokes on back, arms, legs, and abdomen.

- Use fingertips to massage in small circles along baby's body.

- If you're massaging a very young or pre-term baby, be sure to allow for adequate time (at least 15 minutes). A short period of massage can actually be overstimulating to very young infants and should be avoided.

Massaging Your Child

Start by having your child do some deep breathing to relax his muscles and prepare for the massage. Then do the following:

- Place both your hands gently on your child's back so that he can get accustomed to your touch. Some children may prefer that you massage them through their clothes. (If you decide to take this approach, don't use oil or lotion on your hands!)

- Begin by stroking with a long, fluid motion, using a light touch. Start at the nape of the neck and move lower.

- Use a flat, open palm to rub the body.

- You can use fingers to massage smaller places like feet and face.

- A firmer rolling touch can be used for a deeper massage if your child is comfortable with it. You roll a small amount of skin between fingers and thumb, moving up the body. This can be especially relaxing on arms and legs.

Unhappy Baby Alert

Don't press on the spine. Work next to the spine, not on it!

- Try a deeper touch for tight muscles. Use your fingers, thumb, or heel of a hand to press deeper. This technique can be done in a circular motion.

◆ Use these techniques on shoulders, arms, legs, back, and abdomen.

Assorted Health-Giving Practices

A variety of practices related to massage have grown out of the Eastern tradition. They include ...

◆ Acupressure: using touch to unblock energy and heal disease.

◆ Acupuncture: using needles to stimulate the body and unblock energy.

◆ Reflexology: applying pressure to specific points in the feet and hands that correspond with body parts to release energy.

◆ Reiki: energy healing. No direct touch is needed to help relax the body and unblock the body's energy.

The Least You Need to Know

◆ Touch is important to children. Massaging your baby or child can not only help her relax but can make her feel safe and loved.

◆ Practicing yoga exercises can help your child relax and feel ready for bed.

◆ Basic Tai Chi movements can help your child mentally clear his head and calm him physically.

◆ Even your breathing affects how stressed or relaxed you feel. Deep, conscious breathing can help your child feel less stressed and calmer.

Chapter 22

Creating Soothing Environments

In This Chapter

◆ How clearing the clutter can help your child sleep

◆ Creating a calm and peaceful bedroom environment to promote sleep

◆ What the nose knows—using aromatherapy to relax your child

◆ Using music to soothe the savage beast—or at least the crying baby

In this chapter, we'll offer some tried-and-true strategies for creating a soothing environment for your baby or child to sleep in. From aromatherapy to Feng Shui, we've got something for everyone!

Getting Some Rest with Feng Shui

While we won't get into the details (and there are lots), suffice it to say that the principles of *Feng Shui* can be used to help create a soothing sleep environment for your child.

BABY BABBLE

Feng Shui ("fung-schway") is the Chinese art of arranging living spaces to create positive energy, health, and well-being.

Infant Almanac

Don't forget to clear the clutter in other spaces where your child spends a lot of time, such as the family room. This makes your child's home environment more relaxing—and not just for him!

The most important step is to clear the clutter. Physical clutter symbolizes mental clutter. A messy room can make it harder for the child to sleep. Helping your child spend a few minutes cleaning up and putting toys away can make a big difference in the quality of her sleep.

Certified Feng Shui practitioner Mary Mihaly says that you can help create calming energy in a child's room by decorating with Feng Shui principles in mind. Use the following simple guidelines to help your child rest and sleep. According to Mary …

◆ The most common mistake people make is to decorate kids' rooms in stimulating primary colors. Like adults, they need a restful environment if they're going to rest! Soft pastels are best—muted light greens, blues, or a pale yellow all work.

◆ No TV, computer, games, or bookshelves. Although that's very difficult to avoid in many homes, especially when the bedroom is the child's only private space, the computer always beckons with games and e-mail, or distracts from sleep by reminding the child of school projects not yet completed.

◆ A book or two is fine, especially if reading is a sleep-inducer for the child.

◆ Lighting should be soothing—no glaring bare bulbs.

◆ The bed should be in the "command position," which means she can see the door from the bed. This is reassuring to the child. She can see whoever is entering or leaving the room but is not directly in front of the door where she can be easily distracted.

Basically the bed should be as far from the door as possible, facing the room and the door, but not placed so that the child's feet are pointing directly out the door.

♦ No one should sleep under the "low end" of a slanted ceiling. Even it out with a canopy or even an umbrella hanging upside down to symbolize a flat ceiling—but be sure that the umbrella doesn't have a sharp point at the end, pointing at the child's body.

♦ Ceiling beams symbolize knives slashing down, injuring the person and destroying the energy field. They can also be covered with a canopy or at least painted to match the ceiling.

♦ No ceiling fans, if possible; they cut through the energy field while you sleep. (They're okay on very high ceilings.)

♦ Never place the bed in such a way that the child will sleep with his head against a wall containing water pipes; it can flush away his energy, dreams, and good health.

♦ The child's bed needs a headboard to protect energy, dreams, and health from drifting away in the night.

♦ No square corners should be aimed at the child while she's in bed. They direct "sha" or "killing" energy at the sleeping person. If it's necessary to arrange the room with corners aimed at the sleeping person, soften them with a scarf trailing over the corner, a string of silk flowers, or even fresh paint.

♦ The child should not be able to see himself in mirrors when he's reclining in bed.

♦ No dragon images or angry, fierce posters should be hung in the bedroom. They can create negative, hostile energy in the child.

Melissa's Mindset

Research shows that children with a television or computer in their rooms sleep less than those who do not have a media-rich bedroom. Whether or not you're using the principles of Feng Shui to decorate your child's room, keep this in mind.

Using Sounds to Help Baby Sleep

Music—and other sounds—can help lull your baby to sleep for a variety of reasons. Lullabies soothe your baby and remind her of your presence. Nature music calms and relaxes. White noise drowns out other noises that might startle or disturb the baby. Heartbeat recordings remind your baby of the comfort of being in your womb.

Melissa's Mindset

Nickolas still enjoys listening to music to help him sleep. We regularly listen to Enya through the night, but any soft, calming music can work.

All of these sounds can help your baby fall asleep. Some of the sounds can be used even when your child is older, such as white noise and nature music.

Lullabies and Sleepy Time Music

You don't have to have a good singing voice to sing your baby to sleep! She won't care. She'll just be glad to hear the sound of your voice.

We've listed the words to a few lullabies below, but you can find more in books or online. You may also be able to borrow lullaby CDs from the library.

Rock-a-Bye Baby

Rock-a-bye baby, in the tree top
When the wind blows, the cradle will rock
When the bough breaks, the cradle will fall
And down will come baby, cradle and all

Twinkle, Twinkle, Little Star

Twinkle, twinkle, little star
How I wonder what you are!
Up above the world so high
Like a diamond in the sky
Twinkle, twinkle, little star
How I wonder what you are

Hush, Little Baby

This one is also called The Mockingbird Song. Jennifer always changes the "papa" to "mama" when she sings it to Jessica—who at age 8 sometimes still requests it!

Hush, little baby, don't say a word.
Papa's gonna buy you a mockingbird

And if that mockingbird won't sing,
Papa's gonna buy you a diamond ring

And if that diamond ring turns brass,
Papa's gonna buy you a looking glass

And if that looking glass gets broke,
Papa's gonna buy you a billy goat

And if that billy goat won't pull,
Papa's gonna buy you a cart and bull

And if that cart and bull turn over
Papa's going buy you a dog named Rover

And if that dog named Rover won't bark
papa's going buy you a horse and cart

And if that horse and cart fall down
You'll still be the sweetest little baby in town

White Noise

White noise is anything that drowns out other sounds so that they don't startle the person trying to sleep (in this case, your baby or child).

You "listen" to the white noise instead of the other noise (such as people talking in another room, cars zooming down the nearby highway, or the dog barking next door). This way, the other noise doesn't bother you so much, enabling you to fall asleep, or rather enabling your baby or child to fall asleep.

You can use a fan as white noise. Set it on low and face it away from the baby unless you're also using the fan to cool down the room. Remember to use care: an unsupervised child could easily knock a fan over or stick his fingers into the blades. A humidifier works well in providing white noise, too.

Another option is to use a white-noise machine, which is specifically designed to mask ambient sounds. This can be purchased inexpensively at many discount and department stores.

Nature Music

Nature music can also be used to lull your baby or child to sleep. Running water, wind blowing through leaves, crickets chirping, birds cheeping—all of these sounds are soothing to our minds because we're part of nature. They remind us of our connection to the outside world, and soothe our nerves.

Nature music can also drown out other noises, so it can be used the same way white noise is used.

If your baby wakes up in the middle of the night and the music isn't on, she may have trouble falling back to sleep. In that case, you may want to set the CD player on "repeat" or use a continuous-playback tape player.

You can find nature music tapes and CDs at most music stores and at many discount and department stores.

Heartbeat Recordings

You can use a heartbeat recording to help your baby fall asleep. This is less useful for older children. The idea is that the baby is used to hearing his mother's heartbeat (while in the womb) and so letting the baby hear the heartbeat outside of the womb is reassuring. Some studies have shown that listening to a heartbeat recording helps babies fall asleep and cry less.

Almost any rhythmic sound can help comfort a baby, especially if it's coupled with rhythmic moving (such as rocking).

Aromatherapy

You can use smells to help your baby or child relax. Aromatherapy uses the body's sense of smell to change your mood—in this case, to help your baby or child wind down enough to fall asleep.

Lavender is a mild smell that can be very relaxing. Rubbing some lavender body lotion onto a baby's feet can help a fussy baby calm down and get some sleep. You can also use this body lotion to give a massage (see Chapter 21) to an older child. An older child can also sleep with a lavender-scented eye pillow.

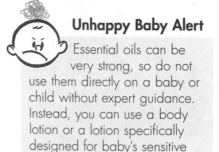

Unhappy Baby Alert

Essential oils can be very strong, so do not use them directly on a baby or child without expert guidance. Instead, you can use a body lotion or a lotion specifically designed for baby's sensitive skin.

To add scent to a room, you can use a plug-in scent dispenser or potpourri (kept out of reach of the child).

The Least You Need to Know

◆ Clearing the clutter and following Feng Shui decorating tips can help your child sleep better.

◆ Listening to all kinds of sounds—lullabies, white noise, nature music, heartbeat recordings—can help your child (especially a young baby) fall asleep.

◆ Lavender helps the body relax and feel ready for sleep.

◆ Creating a soothing bedroom environment can help promote sleep.

Glossary

acupressure   Using firm touch to unblock energy and heal disease.

acupuncture   Using needles to stimulate the body and unblock energy.

affirmations   Positive thoughts you can teach your child to think about as he meditates, such as, "I do well in school," or, "I have good friends and am a good friend." The idea is that instead of listening to the negative, stressful thoughts in his brain, he can create positive affirmations to replace them.

apnea   See *Sleep apnea*.

aromatherapy   Using the body's sense of smell to change your mood.

Attention Deficit-Hyperactivity Disorder (ADHD)   ADHD is the most common psychiatric disorder among children. Common symptoms include difficulty paying attention, distractibility, difficult transitioning from one task to another, and lack of impulse control. Older children may have trouble with being organized and with complex thinking tasks.

baby-led weaning   Relying on the baby to let you know when she is ready to be weaned from any activity that depends on you—nursing, co-sleeping, and so on.

"back to sleep" The phrase to remember when it comes time to put your baby down to sleep. Studies have shown that the risk of Sudden Infant Death Syndrome (SIDS) is dramatically reduced when babies are placed on their backs to sleep.

bedtime routines Comforting bedtime rituals that help your baby realize it's bedtime.

bruxism Medical term for grinding your teeth.

changing your routine When you identify what isn't working, figure out why, and substitute a more successful approach.

checking the baby or child Going into the room to reassure the child, but spending only a few minutes with her.

circadian rhythm The 24-hour biological cycle that governs eating and sleeping, hormonal functions, and other physiological functions.

co-sleeping Sharing your bed with your baby. Goes by many other names: the family bed, bed-sharing, sleep-sharing.

"crying it out" approaches The basic idea behind these approaches is that if you ignore your baby's crying at bedtime, he will learn (eventually) to fall asleep without your intervention. These sleep-training approaches are referred to as "extinction" methods by sleep researchers.

deep sleep Nonrapid eye movement (NREM or non-REM) sleep. Although this type of sleep recurs throughout the night, it's concentrated toward the beginning of nighttime sleep. That's why most night terrors occur in the first couple of hours after the child falls asleep. See Chapter 2 for more information on REM and non-REM sleep.

deformational plagiocephaly A permanently misshapen head, which can occur if the baby doesn't have a sufficient amount of supervised tummy time.

Feng Shui Pronounced "fung schway," it's the Chinese art of arranging living spaces to create positive energy, health, and well-being.

Ferberize To use the "graduated extinction" sleep-training methods of Dr. Richard Ferber to help your baby or child learn to sleep on her own.

Ferber method   An approach to sleep training called "graduated extinction" which requires parents to let the child cry it out for progressively longer periods of time.

growing pains   Unexplained aches and pains that may keep your child up at night, probably related to overexertion.

hypnotherapist   See *Pediatric hypnotherapists.*

"ignore but check" approach   An approach where you create a comforting bedtime routine for your baby or child and then leave him alone, while checking in occasionally—according to a schedule of progressively longer absences—until the child does fall asleep.

"ignore it" approach (or "ignoring/systematic extinction" approach)   An approach that focuses on teaching your child how to fall asleep without your help.

"ignore it but be there" approach   An approach where you stay in the room while doing a full extinction method with your child.

intention   Simply put, the reason you're doing what you're doing. By setting your alarm, you're intending to get up in time for work. Intentions are used to help you (or your child) focus on the purpose for doing a particular relaxation method.

intermittent reinforcement   Responding sometimes—which is the best way to *keep* a behavior happening.

lovey   Technically, "transitional object"—a favorite toy or blanket that comforts the baby. Most babies don't choose a consistent lovey until after the first year of life, but many use a variety of different things (pacifiers, blankets, toys) during the first year.

light sleep   Refers to dreaming or rapid eye movement (REM) sleep. Most dreams occur in this type of sleep, and although periods of REM sleep occur throughout the night, it is concentrated in the early morning hours.

massage   Using touch to stroke, rub, and manipulate the soft tissues of the body to relieve stress and promote health.

narcolepsy   A rare neurological disorder that results in severe daytime sleepiness (the main symptom). Poor sleep, vivid dreams, and sleep paralysis are all symptoms of narcolepsy as is the telltale sign of falling asleep during normal daytime activities.

negative sleep associations Things that won't be there, should your baby wake up in the middle of the night.

Night Owl or Delayed Sleep Phase Syndrome Children with delayed sleep phase syndrome have an internal clock set different from the rest of the world, which means they *can't* go to sleep earlier.

night terror A sleep disorder (known in the sleep world as a "parasomnia") that happens in deep sleep and is characterized by the child sitting upright and screaming about 90 minutes to 2 hours after falling asleep. The child appears to be frightened and is impossible to console.

paradoxical effect Opposite reaction than intended. Generally used to refer to a medication that does the opposite of what it is supposed to do—for example, a sedative that induces hyperactive behavior in some children.

pediatric hypnotherapists Clinicians who teach children how to self-hypnotize and can show you how to help your child with the method.

periodic breathing Occasional pauses in a baby's breathing that may last up to 10 seconds, related to a newborn's immature respiratory system. It takes a while for breathing responses (and the muscles involved in breathing) to develop in infants. Many parents are alarmed by periodic breathing for fear that it may be apnea. Generally speaking, the pause should last less than 10 seconds. If it lasts more than 10 seconds, your baby may have apnea. Consult a pediatrician if you're at all concerned.

"persistent gentle removal system" approach This approach is used to eliminate night wakings by changing the sleep associations your infant has. For example, babies who are rocked to sleep have trouble soothing themselves from night wakings without parental intervention, so this approach will require you to change your ways.

polysomnography A recording done (usually at a sleep center) that measures brain waves, heart rate, muscle tone, and the like, in order to help diagnose sleep disorders.

postpartum depression A serious, persistent, negative mental state (worse than the "blues") that may occur after the birth of a child.

postpartum psychosis An extreme but rare form of depression after the birth of a child, involving hallucinations and delusions.

proactive co-sleeping When parents plan and enjoy the practice of bed-sharing.

reactive co-sleeping When parents react to sleep problems in their children by sharing the same bed out of desperation.

reflexology Applying pressure to specific points in the feet and hands that correspond with body parts, to release energy.

Reiki Energy healing. No direct touch is needed to help relax the body and unblock the body's energy.

Restless Legs Syndrome A disorder that causes an uncomfortable feeling in the legs, causing the child affected to toss and turn and have difficulty falling asleep.

"scheduled awakenings" approach This method is used for babies and children who do not have a problem settling at bedtime, but do wake frequently through the night. Using this method, you put the baby to bed at bedtime, using whatever approach you have chosen to encourage her to fall asleep by herself, then awaken her shortly before her typical night waking times. Because she'll be tired, she will fall back to sleep within a few minutes and probably will not have an unscheduled awakening. Over time, this method may help extinguish night wakings.

self-hypnosis A method of creating focused concentration in your mind; can also be a method you can use to learn to relax your body.

self-soothing The ability of a baby or child to comfort himself after waking without requiring parental presence (by feeding, rocking, and so on).

sidecar method Using a crib-type bed that attaches to your bed. The baby sleeps next to you but is less vulnerable to overlying, wedging, and other dangers. In addition to a sidecar-style bassinet that attaches to the bed, a mini-bassinet now on the market can be placed on the mattress. It has small sides that keep the baby separate from parents and prevent overlying.

sidelying Sometimes pediatricians recommend sidelying (putting baby to bed on her side) for babies who spit up a lot. Make sure you understand exactly how to position your baby if this is recommended for you. If this has not been specifically recommended, keep baby on her back for sleep.

sleep apnea   Breathing cessation during sleep. It is a sleep disorder that should be treated by a physician.

sleep associations   Objects and activities that your baby connects with falling asleep.

sleep consolidation   The process during which babies begin sleeping for longer consecutive periods of time and mostly at night.

sleep-disordered breathing   See *sleep apnea*.

sleep hygiene   Good sleep habits that ensure that your baby eventually learns to fall asleep on his own and can soothe himself back to sleep after night wakings.

sleep training   Using specific strategies to help your baby learn to fall asleep by herself at bedtime and to fall back to sleep when she wakes during the night.

sleeping through the night   People define "sleeping through the night" in different ways. Some consider midnight to 4 A.M. as sleeping through the night. This is important for parents to keep in mind when considering the claims made by supporters of different sleep-training approaches.

"splitting it up" approach   This approach uses steps similar to the "ignore but check" method, sometimes called the Ferber method, described in Chapter 7—letting the child fuss for progressively longer periods of time—but you don't deal with bedtime and night wakings at the same time. This means you're stricter about how you handle bedtime, and more flexible about how you respond to nighttime wakings—at first. Later, you deal with night wakings more systematically if you need to.

spontaneous awakenings   Waking that the baby does on his own without your help. The goal of the "scheduled awakenings" approach is to get rid of the spontaneous awakenings.

Sudden Infant Death Syndrome (SIDS)   The sudden and unexplained death of a baby under the age of one, after a postmortem examination and review of the infant's medical history.

swaddling   Snugly wrapping your baby in a blanket for warmth and security.

Tai Chi (or Taiji)   An ancient Chinese martial art that is based on Taoist philosophy. Tai Chi encourages a supple, flexible mind, body, and spirit. Tai Chi movements can be used to help relax and settle the body and mind in time for bed.

transitional object   A favorite toy, stuffed animal, or blanket a young child can use to comfort herself while falling asleep and throughout the night (instead of relying on you to provide the comfort).

verbal contact   Using words to soothe the baby rather than picking him up, nursing him, and so on. "Mama's here," "Hush, baby, time for sleep," and the like, let the baby know you're there but encourage him to fall asleep without more active intervention from you.

"wait it out" approach   An approach where you and the rest of the family hunker down and put up with some nighttime challenges, hoping that your baby will outgrow her problems and eventually organize her sleep so that everyone can get a little shut-eye.

white noise   Noise or sound that drowns out other sounds so that they don't startle the baby.

yoga   An Eastern practice that encourages health and well-being. Practitioners move their bodies into various "poses" that help stretch the body, work joints, and stimulate muscles.

Appendix B

Resources

If you need a little help on your sleep-training quest, this is the place to start.

Sounds to Sleep By

"The Heartbeat CD" is a recording of a regular heartbeat to help baby sleep. www.heartbeatcd.com

"Infant Calm" is a collection of six household sounds (e.g., "white noise") that calms colicky/fussy babies. www.prerecords.com

"Storieszzz: The Adventures of Faye & Fred" are four original short stories that will relax your child and help her fall asleep. www.prerecords.com

"Night Night Time" and other lullaby collections. www.sleeplullabies.com

"Journey into Sleep: Hypnosis for Power Naps and Deep Rest" is a relaxation CD created by a hypnotherapist. www.whiteheartpublishing.com or www.amazon.com

Yoga and Tai Chi

The Power of Relaxation: Using Tai Chi and Visualization to Reduce Children's Stress. Book by Patrice Thomas. Redleaf Press, 2005. ISBN: 1-929610-378. www.redleafpress.org

Tai Chi for Kids: Move with the Animals. Book for children ages 4–8 by Stuart Alve Olson. Bear Cub Books, 2001. ISBN: 1-879181-657. www.amazon.com

David Carradine's A.M. and P.M. Tai Chi Workout for Beginners. DVD. www.amazon.com

Itsy Bitsy Yoga: Poses to Help Your Baby Sleep Longer, Digest Better, and Grow Stronger. Book by Helen Garabedian. Fireside, 2001. ISBN: 0-743242-552. www.amazon.com

Yoga Kids. A series of DVDs encouraging children to do yoga. www.amazon.com

For more information and to find a teacher, check out this website: www.childrensyoga.com

Hypnosis

For more information about hypnosis, try these websites:

The University of Michigan health-care system www.med.umich.edu/1libr/yourchild/hypnosis.htm

An organization that sells hypnosis CDs and services: www.NewBehaviorInstitute.net

The website of the American Society of Clinical Hypnosis: www.asch.net

Sleep Centers

If you're concerned that your baby or child may have a sleep disorder or you feel you need more help with his sleep problems, look into getting help from a sleep center or pediatric sleep specialist.

The center should be accredited by the AASM (American Academy of Sleep Medicine) and should have at least one pediatric specialist who is certified by the AASM—pediatrician, pulmonologist, psychiatrist, neurologist, or psychologist.

The first step is to find an accredited center. Then, contact the center to see if they have a certified pediatric specialist on staff.

Visit www.sleepcenters.org to find a list of accredited sleep centers.

Index

s

crib bed transition, 172-173
family bed transition,
171-172

S

Sadeh, Avi, *Sleeping Like a Baby*,
107
safety, 5-6, 9
co-sleeping method, 129-131
scheduled awakenings method,
106
advantages, 112
approach supporters, 107
basics, 106-107
disadvantages, 112
following approach, 107
challenges, 111-112
controlling waking times,
108-110
troubleshooting, 110-111
parents' opinions, 113
schedules
eliminating chaos, 7
ignore but be there method,
87-89
ignore but feed method, 77-79
ignore it method, 64
persistent gentle removal
system method, 142
schoolagers
approach modification, 190
creating bedtime routine,
186-187
resistance problems, 187-188
trouble falling asleep,
188-189
waking up, 188
reasons for sleep problems,
178-179
bedwetting, 183-184
medical conditions, 185-186
napping, 180
nightmares, 180-181

night terrors, 181-182
sleeptalking, 184-185
sleepwalking, 184-185
selecting effective sleep
method, 189
schools, start time adjustments,
195
Sears, Dr. Williams, 127
Sears, Martha, 127
secondhand smoke, sleep apnea
connection, 24
self-hypnosis. *See* hypnosis
self-soothing, 4, 75
severe developmental delays, 209
side sleeping, 5
SIDS (Sudden Infant Death
Syndrome)
apnea risks, 24
sleep safety, 5
six-month-olds, sleep development, 21-22
Sleep Baby Sleep, 138
sleep
babies' needs, 17
consolidation, 21
cycles, babies, 14-15
deprivation, 30-31
older children, 193
parents, 52
signs, 193-194
development, 19-20, 31
adolescents, 33-34
children with special needs,
34
gradeschoolers, 33
newborns, 20
nine-month-olds, 22
one-year-olds, 22-23
preschoolers, 32-33
six-month-olds, 21-22
three-month-olds, 21
disorders, 24, 35
disruptions
babies, 22-25

Check Out These
Best-Sellers

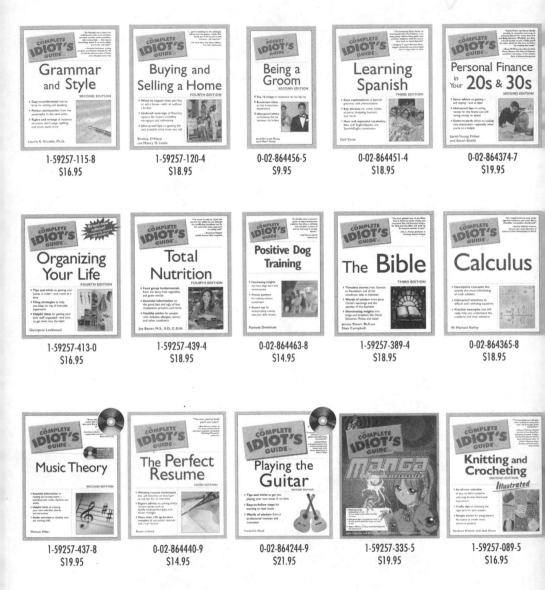

Grammar and Style SECOND EDITION	**Buying and Selling a Home** FOURTH EDITION	**Being a Groom**	**Learning Spanish** THIRD EDITION	**Personal Finance in Your 20s & 30s** SECOND EDITION
1-59257-115-8 $16.95	1-59257-120-4 $18.95	0-02-864456-5 $9.95	0-02-864451-4 $18.95	0-02-864374-7 $19.95
Organizing Your Life FOURTH EDITION	**Total Nutrition** FOURTH EDITION	**Positive Dog Training**	**The Bible** THIRD EDITION	**Calculus**
1-59257-413-0 $16.95	1-59257-439-4 $18.95	0-02-864463-8 $14.95	1-59257-389-4 $18.95	0-02-864365-8 $18.95
Music Theory SECOND EDITION	**The Perfect Resume** THIRD EDITION	**Playing the Guitar** SECOND EDITION	**Manga Illustrated**	**Knitting and Crocheting** SECOND EDITION Illustrated
1-59257-437-8 $19.95	0-02-864440-9 $14.95	0-02-864244-9 $21.95	1-59257-335-5 $19.95	1-59257-089-5 $16.95

More than *450 titles* available at booksellers and online retailers everywhere

www.idiotsguides.com

ALPHA